PILATES
PERFECT

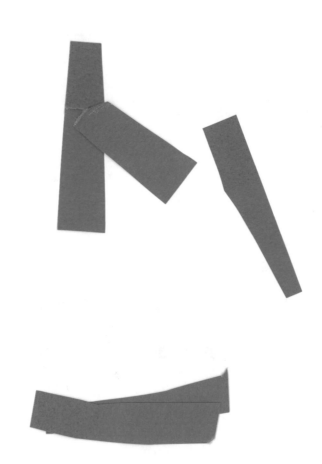

PILATES
PERFECT

THE COMPLETE GUIDE TO PILATES EXERCISE AT HOME

DIANNE DANIELS, MA
Photographs by Peter Field Peck

CPL

healthyliving**books**
New York • London

A HEALTHY LIVING BOOK
Hatherleigh Press
5-22 46th Avenue, Suite 200
Long Island City, NY 11101
Visit our Web site:
www.healthylivingbooks.com

Library of Congress Cataloging-in-Publication Data

Daniels, Dianne.
  Pilates perfect : the complete guide to pilates exercise at home : improve
your posture, increase your flexibility, flatten your abs, boost your energy
/ Dianne Daniels ; photographs by Peter Field Peck.
      p. cm.
  ISBN 1-57826-147-3
  1. Pilates method. I. Title.
  RA781.4.D36 2004
  613.7'1--dc22
                              2004014898

HEALTHY LIVING BOOKS are available for bulk purchase, special promotions, and premiums. For information on reselling and special purchase opportunities, please call us at 1-800-528-2550 and ask for the Special Sales Manager.

Cover and interior design by Tai Blanche
Photographs by Peter Field Peck

10 9 8 7 6 5 4 3 2
Printed in Canada

Dedication

To all my students and all my teachers—past, present, and future.

With Appreciation

To all the talented people who participated in the thinking, creating, editing, and layout of this book, and especially to Mary Beltran for her overwhelming generosity of time and ideas, and to my models, Jen Howard and Andrew Flach, for their great spirit and boundless energy.

Table of Contents

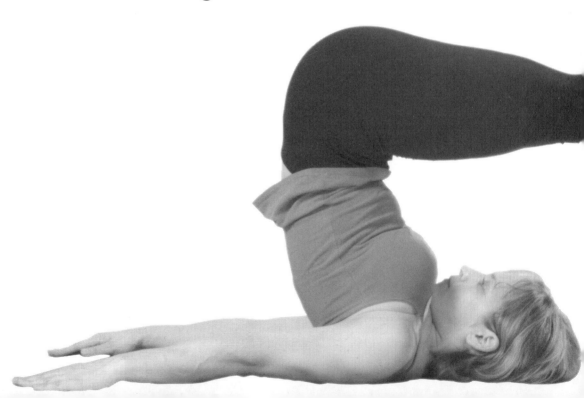

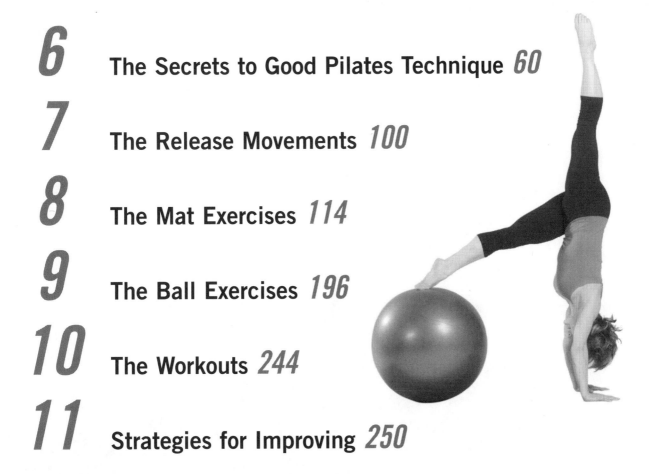

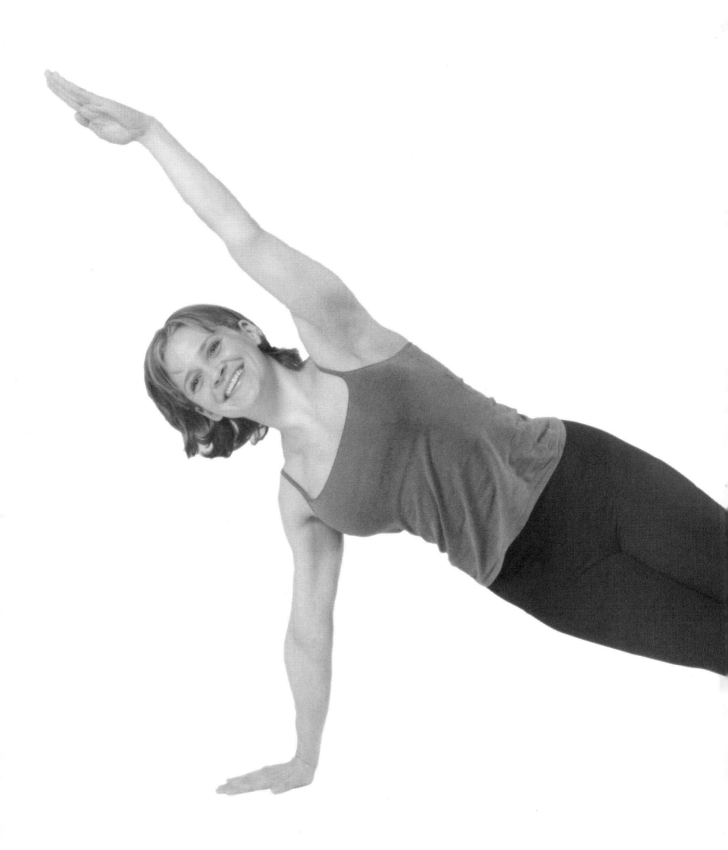

Why *This* Pilates Book is Different

Y ou're probably wondering what, if anything, makes *this* Pilates book different from all the others on the shelf next to it. Well, it's full of creative shortcuts to help you achieve the grace and power that is the embodiment of the Pilates program. If you ever wanted to attain that Pilates "look," with toned abdominals and a strong back, these innovative ideas will guide you to the improved appearance and greater health you're probably seeking if you've picked up this book. Not only will you learn how to do Pilates exercises correctly and safely, you will soon be able to do them with more ease, comfort, and enjoyment.

The shortcuts you will learn in this book are unique and highly effective. They combine Pilates with a movement reeducation approach called The Feldenkrais Method®. This synthesis was designed by me, and has my students loving every minute of the classes I teach.

Over the years, as I looked around the room at my students, I marveled at their commitment to conquering the demands of the method. Yet despite the best of efforts and the fiercest devotion, some could never overcome muscular or skeletal impediments. Knees and elbows were always bent and it was impossible to completely straighten them; sitting in good, upright posture was an uncomfortable experience; legs or feet would cramp. It was a strain to hold the head or legs off the floor for an extended time. Bodies simply would not acquiesce to what they were being asked to do. Still, they persevered; because of how much better they felt after the workout; because aches and pains would disappear; because they awakened with a new sense of power.

Here's how this Pilates book stands apart from the rest: It teaches you how to surpass your present capabilities to achieve what you never dreamed was within your grasp. As an exercise physiologist with a fitness orientation and a breadth of hands-on experience, I know how to make an impossible exercise possible. On almost every page is an exercise option that suits your current abilities and one to meet your future aspirations.

To keep the workouts fresh and exciting, I've gone beyond the traditional Pilates workout to include exercises that have evolved from the method. You'll find that your body, as well as your mind, will be continually stimulated from this diverse collection for many years to come.

Firming the abdominals, strengthening the back, toning the arms and sculpting the legs are only a small part of the Pilates story. The *how* it is done is what evolves into the visual and internal changes that affect your posture, your strength, your flexibility, and the spring in your step.

A
word
of
caution

It is imperative that you
consult your physician before
you embark on this, or any,
exercise program. Pilates is strenuous
exercise and not suitable for everyone.
This book is not intended as advice or assurance to any specific reader regarding his or her
ability to perform this program safely.

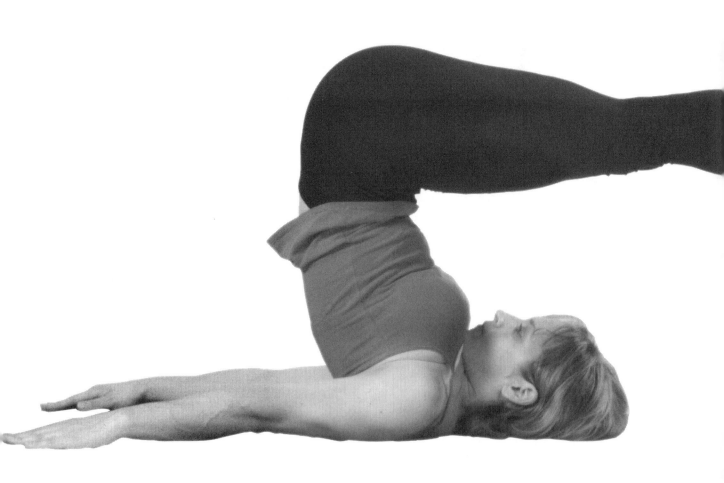

Chapter 1

Pilates Perfect Is for Everyone

Transformation Awaits

Strength. Vigor. Control. Intensity. Energy. We all aspire to cultivate these, and other characteristics commonly associated with power. They are also the beneficial outcomes from consistent and faithful Pilates practice.

Young or old, athlete or couch potato, or somewhere in between, Pilates has a role to play as you seek to develop a lifetime habit of exercising wisely and successfully. Once learned, the essential elements of Pilates can be yours forever, to take with you as you stay active and pursue other fitness interests.

An Unbeatable Combination: Strength and Flexibility

Pilates is a whole body exercise program that simultaneously strengthens *and* lengthens your muscles. Many begin doing Pilates to get toned abdominals; it will certainly do that. The traditional "ab work" you may have participated in at a gym or health club cannot compare to what Pilates has to offer. Say goodbye to doing hundreds of crunches. Get ready to embrace a program that is diverse, challenging, and exciting.

A Unique Approach

Pilates is powerful exercise because it uses the mind to improve the body. Your focus, concentration, and attention are called upon with every movement. Without this mental aspect fully engaged you would simply be doing movements; you would not be doing Pilates.

It takes power to involve your whole self with each exercise. Each part of your body will be called upon to move, or *not* to move. Surprisingly, it will be this movement *inhibition* that will be your greatest challenge, taking weeks and months of practice to attain, and years to perfect.

You will gain even more insight into your body's capabilities through the powerful pairing of Pilates with gentle movements inspired by the Feldenkrais method. It will feel as though someone has squirted lubricant directly into your joints. Movements will feel smoother, easier, lighter, and more pleasant. Your body will respond to you—it will do what you want it to—and you will find your skill level increasing quickly.

It Won't Take Long to Reap the Benefits

Happily, part of the power of Pilates is that it gives you almost immediate benefits, regardless of your fitness level or where you are in the program's progression. You can expect to feel and see changes within a matter of weeks. Your abdominal area will feel firmer. Your arms and legs will begin to attain a toned appearance. You'll feel taller and lighter when you walk. Chronic discomforts will disappear. That nagging back problem, the shoulder irritation, chronic hip pain—gone.

Each time you do the program, you will come away feeling energized, renewed, and looking forward to your next session.

A "New" Workout, With a History

Joseph Pilates was born in Germany in 1880. A frail child, he developed this program of exercise to build himself up. Since its introduction to America in 1926, the Pilates method has acquired a devout following. But it is only within the last few years that it has experienced a surge of popularity, making it a hot "new" fitness trend. Today, because more and more exercise enthusiasts are savvy enough to know when they are getting a good exercise "product," Pilates is seeing a substantial jump in the number of students taking part in its rigorous training.

Pilates has gone mainstream since it was first discovered by dancers and professional athletes to facilitate performance or rehabilitate from injury. You'll find mat classes in gyms, health clubs, and studios everywhere. If you live in an area where you have the ability to choose a class from several that are available, I suggest you take a look at Chapter 11: *Strategies for Improving,* for ideas on how to judge the quality of a class.

Would You Like to Build Some Bone?

A small, but growing, body of research has shed light on the ability of Pilates and Feldenkrais, each individually, to increase bone density. Imagine, then, how potentially powerful combining them might be.

With osteoporosis plaguing ten percent of the American population and projections suggesting it will become an epidemic in a few years, it's exciting to learn of an exercise strategy that works, and that can be practiced by just about anyone. (If you're interested in beginning an osteoporosis-fighting exercise program, you may want to read my book, *Exercises for Osteoporosis, Revised Edition*, Hatherleigh Press, 2004).

If you have osteoporosis, be sure to consult with your doctor to find the right exercise sequence for you. Seek out the exercises in this book with the stated purpose of back strengthening, as these can be among the most beneficial. Remember to start with the Beginner exercises. To avert a potential bone fracture, avoid the Ball exercises, as it's common to lose your balance and fall from time to time.

It Will Surprise You

If you've never exercised before, or if you're bored with your present exercise regimen, Pilates will open up new vistas. Whether you know little about exercise, or think you know it all, get ready for a revelation.

Chapter 2

How Pilates Changes Your Body

Brain to Brawn

Pilates changes the body from the inside out. The key to success is using your mind as well as your body. In Pilates you won't tune out. Instead, every movement, every repetition, is performed with concentration and mental control. You will learn to tune in to exactly what your body is doing and not doing, what is moving and what is not moving.

Your body will gain new wisdom. What begins as a thought or visualization in your mind is relayed via new neuromuscular connections that trigger your muscles to respond. Sometimes the muscles are called upon to make movements that, though almost imperceptible to the eye, are the very essence of the work.

Getting to the Core

The *core* refers to the muscles that encircle your body's midsection. There are four muscles along the front that comprise what we commonly call "the abdominals." Sometimes they are mischaracterized as "upper" and "lower" abdominals, but a quick review of anatomy reveals the true story.

The muscle closest to the surface is the *rectus abdominus*, which extends from the bottom of the breastbone to the pubic bone. When this muscle contracts, the breastbone and pubic bone will move closer to one another. It is physiologically impossible to separate the "upper" part of this muscle from the "lower" part; it is all one muscle. Sometimes it is possible to target more fibers of either the upper or lower part of the *rectus abdominus*; but keep in mind that when a muscle contracts, the *entire* length of the muscle is involved in the movement.

In the next layer are the *internal* and *external obliques*, which cross the front and back of the body like a corset. Most people are unaware that the obliques actually wrap around the body and insert into a layer of *fascia*, or connective tissue, in the back. Looking still deeper we find the *transverse abdominus*, so named because its muscle fibers run horizontally across the front of the body, from the lower ribs to the top of the hip bone.

Turning to the side and posterior (back) segments, we have the *quadratus lumborum* and *erector spinae*, muscles that support upright posture and facilitate your ability to lift your body from a prone (face down) position.

In summary, the core consists of muscles in the center of your body that encompass your front, sides, and back.

Would You Like a Flat Belly?

In contrast to the traditional abdominal crunches and curls normally seen in gyms and health clubs, Pilates accesses the deepest layer of the abdominal wall, the *transverse abdominus*. This muscle has the primary responsibility of "holding in" an array of organs all vying for a little breathing room in a small cavity. Without a strong *transverse abdominus*, these organs, with nowhere else to go, tend to push forward and create that bulging stomach we all dread so much. This becomes especially apparent as we get older. It's quite common to see an otherwise thin elderly person with a protruding stomach, which is the ultimate manifestation of the scenario described above.

As you pay close attention to the instructions for each exercise you will most likely find a total overhaul of your usual technique is necessary. Instead of pulling on your neck, using momentum to propel your body up, tucking your pelvis under, pushing your stomach forward, or engaging other muscles to assist, you will be *isolating* just the abdominals to do the work. This will greatly curtail the number of repetitions you will be able to do. In fact, a person who can perform hundreds of abdominal curls is probably using accessory muscles and not truly isolating the abdominals.

With correct execution of the Pilates exercises, each and every repetition will engage the *transverse abdominus*, the most powerful muscle in your quest for the perfect mid-section.

Staying Free of Injury

A person with a strong *core* has a powerful corset of muscles to actively support the spine and help protect it from harm.

Do you know someone who is constantly throwing out his or her back? They've probably lifted something, made a sudden turn, or perhaps bent over—all movements requiring either strength or flexibility of the spine. (By the way, did you know back pain is the number one reason people miss work?) There are myriad reasons for back pain and if you experience it you should have it evaluated by a physician. If the condition can be remedied through exercise, Pilates might be recommended as the exercise program of choice.

The single most important factor creating susceptibility to injury is probably *muscular imbalance*. These inequalities occur in your body even from a young age. At first they are pain free; with the advancement of years, however, they may begin to take a toll on your body.

Here's an example of what I'm talking about. Stand in front of a mirror and look at yourself closely. Unless you're one in a million, you'll see that one shoulder is higher than the other (perhaps ever so slightly, perhaps quite a lot). This unevenness has already been transmitted throughout your body, making it necessary for your torso to compensate by bending a little more to the left or right, for your pelvis to make a shift, perhaps for the thigh bone to rotate—all the way down to which part of your foot bears your body's weight.

Our bodies are comprised of "matched sets"—we have two of almost every muscle, one on the right and one on the left. One side can become more *hypertrophied* (bigger) than the other because of *how* we use our bodies. Don't assume that if you're right or left handed this means one entire side of your body will be stronger than the other. Each muscle pairing is unique, with its own history of how it has been used, or abused, over the years.

Let's say that you habitually raise or hunch up your shoulders as you're about to do something that requires effort, even if it's just a slight effort that's needed. If this becomes a normal pattern you may, as time progresses, begin to experience chronic neck or shoulder aches. Why? Perhaps because the way your shoulder blades are positioned has changed, or your ribs have acquired a new orientation, or you're holding your head tilted at a slightly different angle. Over time habits are etched into your body, laying the groundwork for future injuries or chronic discomforts.

Fortunately, the person who regularly engages in Pilates knows that they are strong enough to meet any challenge. By consistently working toward engaging *all* your body's muscles, Pilates keeps your body in harmony so that you stay strong, healthy, and injury free.

The Changes You Can Expect

Because the Pilates program is so inclusive, the benefits are far reaching. Here's a partial list of the improvements you can expect to attain with consistent practice:

- better posture
- standing taller
- feeling lighter
- longer, leaner muscles
- improved breathing
- more energy
- a flexible spine
- new suppleness throughout your body
- greater ability to focus and concentrate
- improved self-esteem and a sense of personal power

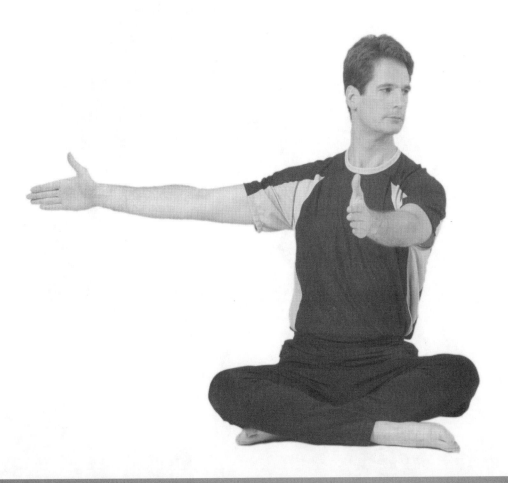

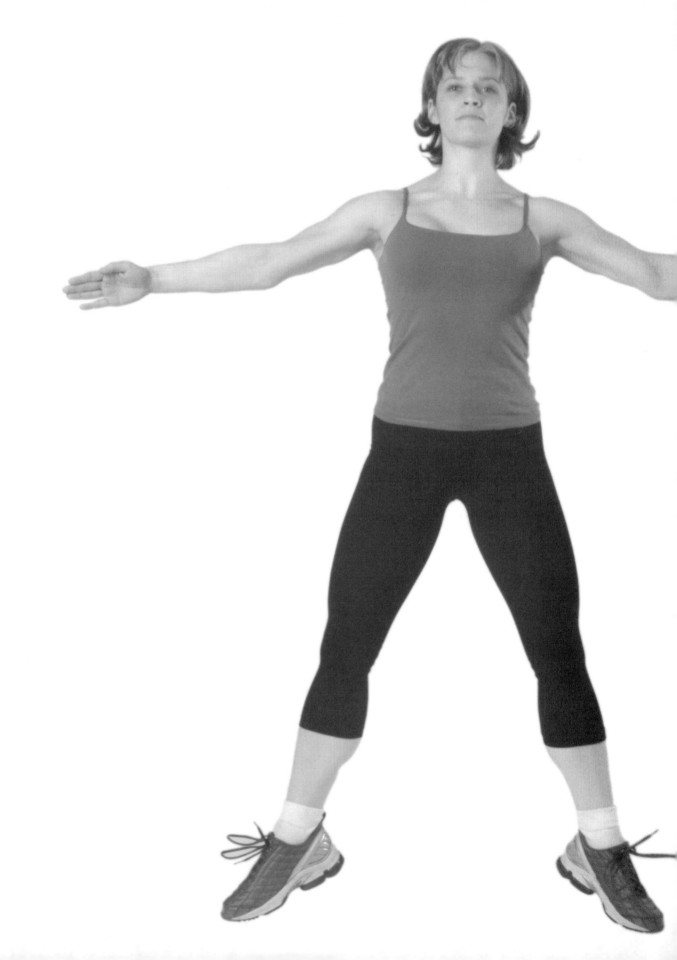

Preparing for the Workout

Start Out on the Right Foot

As is always the advice with any exercise program, consult your doctor to make sure Pilates is appropriate for you. If you have any medical conditions or orthopedic restrictions, this caveat is of special importance. Pilates, done without strict adherence to technique, or advanced too quickly, can cause injuries or harm to your body. On the other hand, Pilates is often recommended by health professionals for rehabilitation purposes, especially for people with chronic back pain or those who have suffered a back injury. When done correctly, Pilates offers relief and recovery.

How to Use This Book

Start with the next chapter, *Learning the Basics.* Each Pilates mat or ball exercise incorporates one or more of these principles. The guiding principles of Pilates are described there and whether you're a beginner or advanced exerciser, need to be practiced thoroughly. Review them often—over time you will gain a richer understanding of what they mean and an improved ability to perform them.

There are many reasons why form and alignment are very important, as you will discover in Chapter 5. There you will learn how to position your body from head to toe. Because Pilates is a *whole* body program, *every* part of your body participates *all* the time, whether or not it is visibly moving. Your neck, shoulders, back, abdominals, legs, toes, arms, fingers, and your breathing, all have a role to play in every Pilates exercise.

Progress to Chapter 6 to learn the *Secrets to Good Pilates Technique* and take a giant step toward attaining that Pilates look. Return to the chapter often to develop the ease, fluidity, flexibility, and range of motion that keeps elevating your performance quality to a higher level.

Because the potential intensity of each exercise is great, you will want to review the *Release Movements* in Chapter 7 that give your muscles the opportunity to rest, recuperate, and lengthen.

You'll begin to feel and see tremendous improvements with practice of the fundamentals in these four chapters alone. When you feel the principles have been instilled in you, move on to the *Mat Exercises* in Chapter 8. And when you've mastered the Mat, it's time to tackle Chapter 9: *The Ball Exercises,* which pose new challenges even for the advanced exerciser.

Workouts are in Chapter 10, and there's where you'll find a program to meet your fitness level and goals.

Are you looking to maximize your new commitment to Pilates, or want to further explore the wonders of Feldenkrais? Then read Chapter 11: *Strategies For Improving,* for ideas worth pursuing.

Mind Over Matter

If you simply repeat the movements in a rote manner, without being attentive to what your body is doing, then you're not doing Pilates.

Be forewarned: If you feel an exercise is easy, that's a sure sign that you are *not* adhering strictly to the instructions. You are most likely neglecting to fully stabilize and engage your muscles correctly. It is always possible to work deeper and harder, to become more attuned to and have greater control over the internal happenings in your body. Pilates, done correctly, will always feel challenging.

Warm Muscles Work Best

Before you start your Pilates routine, do a warm-up so that your muscles are ready to be stretched and strengthened. Muscles work best when they are warm; that is, when the temperature inside the muscles is elevated.

Do a standard aerobics routine or be creative. Put on some music and do the jig, the rumba, or some hip hop dancing. If you're a walker, walk. If you're a stairclimber, then climb. It doesn't matter what you do as long as you feel your body is heating up, that you're beginning to perspire, and that you feel loose and primed to engage your body and your mind to its full potential.

An Easy At-Home Warm Up

Are you without a regular aerobic activity? Then try any or all of these simple moves. You may want to do each 5 or 10 times in sequence, and then start at the top and repeat the sequence again. Whatever your format, your goal is to keep moving for at least five minutes.

1 March in place

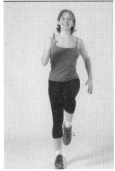

2 Step touches

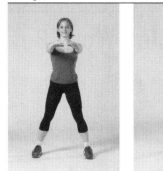

3 Knee lifts

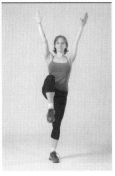

4 Hamstring curls

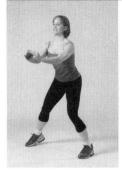
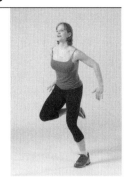

5 Squats

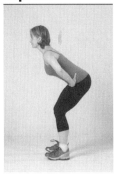

6 Squat with adduction

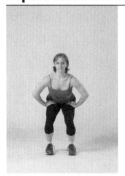
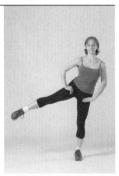

7 **Squat with knee lift**

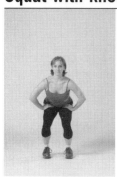 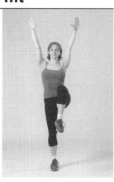

8 **Squat with kick back**

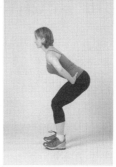 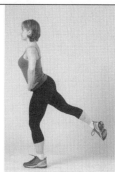

9 **Pliés**

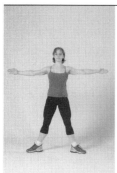 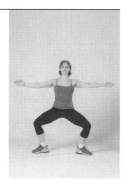

10 **Jumping jacks**

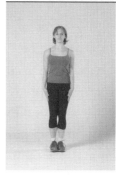 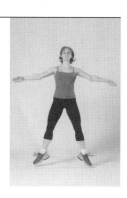

11 **Jumping rope**

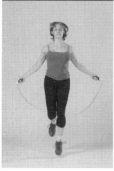

12 **Punching / boxing**

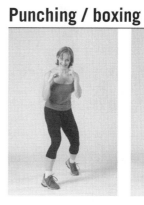 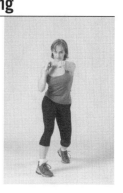

13 **The Rockettes' kicks**

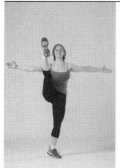

The Details Matter

Let's take a look at the instructions you'll be receiving as you go along, all of which are important for your comfort and safety. They must be incorporated without fail, every time you exercise.

Don't be surprised if at first the instructions seem overwhelming. If you have carefully studied Chapter 4: *Learning the Basics*, you are certainly ready to proceed. The rest is a matter of practice and familiarity with the material. Pilates will always be a work in progress.

Purpose of Exercise

In every Pilates exercise the intention is to fully engage the abdominals to strengthen the core. There are generally additional goals, such as increased strength, toning, or flexibility of a particular muscle or muscle group. Oftentimes these co-existing objectives call for *isometric* strengthening, or stationary holding. For example, if you put yourself in the traditional push-up position and lift and lower your right leg, your chest and arm muscles are working *isometrically* to keep your upper body supported. Your right leg muscles, on the other hand, are working *isotonically*, that is, you actually see movement occurring.

This coordination of your breathing, core, upper and lower body, each with a different function and purpose in a particular exercise, is why Pilates cannot be learned in a day, in a week, or even in a month.

Level

Always start with the Beginner exercises. You will avoid injury and achieve a steady rate of progress by taking it nice and easy and not trying to do too much too soon.

Use your common sense in choosing exercises that are appropriate for your fitness level. *Most advanced exercises should not be attempted if you have a back problem.* Stay at lower levels and, over time, as your back strengthens, you will be able to gradually increase intensity.

Prerequisites

You are referred to a Basic, Mat, or Ball exercise that you should be capable of doing before proceeding. This will both ensure your safety and give you enhanced ability to perform the exercise. For example, you must be able to do the exercise Flight before you attempt Swim, or if you cannot do Leg Pull Back on the mat, don't attempt to do it on the ball.

Enhancements

Improved performance—greater ease, fluidity, increased range of motion—have their genesis in Chapter 6: *The Secrets to Good Pilates Technique*. You may find doing the enhancement just once is all you need to make a difficult exercise smooth and graceful. On the other hand, you may need to repeat these enhancements many times when you begin a specific exercise, until your body spontaneously learns to incorporate these new strategies.

Starting Position

Here's where you'll learn how to position your physical body. Even at the very outset of your Pilates workout program you will begin having an internal conversation with yourself. You will learn how to scan your body for unnecessary tension, align yourself from head to fingers to toes, and explore how and where to lengthen.

Action

You'll be guided through a step-by-step description of the movement or movements that make up each exercise.

Pay strict attention to the instructions. Any exercise can be potentially dangerous, especially if performed incorrectly or too quickly. Move slowly, with control. Avoid jerking, pulling on, or hurling your body.

Before you even begin to move a muscle form an *intention* in your mind. For a moment, think about doing the exercise with a body that's light, flexible, and responsive. It will relax your muscles and offset the tendency to tense up. Try it. It's a very powerful technique.

Breathing cues are included. With each *inhale* breathe in deeply as you imagine a lengthening occurring in your body (reach through your fingers and your legs, feel that the space between each vertebra increase, get taller). And with each *exhale* expel the air completely through pursed lips as you contract your abdominals and perform a Kegel (see page 40).

Repetitions

This is the number of times an exercise should be repeated, or as will be the case for stretches, how long to stay in one position. You can feel free to do fewer. What is important is that you pay strict attention to form. If you can only do one repetition in good form—wonderful. Many repetitions done incorrectly are simply worthless.

Pilates is not a discipline that promotes multiple repetitions of each exercise. You will come to appreciate how variety is used to challenge and surprise the body so it learns to recruit muscles and stabilize the skeleton from various angles and in differing positions. And whatever position you are in—on your stomach, your back, your side, or supported on your hands and toes—you will be working your abdominals.

Body Checks

Take the time to read and re-read these tips often so that you always keep them in mind as you execute the exercise. How can you tell whether you are doing an exercise correctly? You'll find the answer there.

Keep in mind that *where* you are feeling the work of the exercise is crucial; this should *always* be in your abdominals. Can you sense a continual build up of intensity, perhaps that of a burning sensation, in your abdominal area? Regardless of what part of your body is being asked to lift, bend, extend or twist, the effort is always to be centered in, and emanate from, your core.

As *every* part of your body participates in *every* exercise, it's difficult even for the experienced Pilates student to remember it all. Constant, repeated reminders and cueing are an integral part of the teaching strategy, whether you take a live Pilates class, or do your program from a book. You will need to develop a Pilates mantra, a running commentary in your head, to focus constant attention on your form.

Power It Down

If performing the exercise makes you strain your body, use this modification. I promise you will still reap substantial benefits while continuing to work within your zone of safety. You may be given the option to keep your knees bent, to do one repetition and then rest, or to do just a portion of the exercise.

Power It Up

It's always a good feeling when you notice your fitness level has improved. Now you're ready to up the intensity. You may be directed to make the movements bigger, or you might be asked to use a piece of equipment. These include wrist weights, ankle weights, a body bar, or the Magic Ring. If weights are called for, start with the lightest you can find and progressively increase by small increments over a period of days, weeks, and months. The safest plan would be to first use 1/2 pound weights, then progress to 1 pound, then 1 1/2 pounds and so on. Body bars generally begin at 3 pounds, then 6 pounds, 9 pounds, and up from there.

Your Equipment Portfolio

What makes both Pilates and Feldenkrais (which you will learn more about shortly) so powerful is that they require no equipment whatsoever. Certainly if you are a beginner there is no need to use any of the toys that are pictured in this book. However, if you are a long-time exerciser who wants to put a little more zest or novelty in your program, or if there is a particular area of your body that you would like to improve (say more toning for the back of your arms or inner thighs), then you may want to consider the purchase of one or more of the following.

The *Magic Ring* can be used effectively by anyone regardless of fitness level. Its most significant advantage is that it helps with learning how to achieve a Deep Abdominal Contraction. If you're having any difficulty feeling intensity in the abdominal area, then consider adding this piece of equipment to your fitness arsenal. The Magic Ring is also perfect for toning the inner thigh muscles.

The *body bar* is used in this book concurrently to tone the arms and increase exercise intensity. You'll see it only in the *Power It Up* section. If you are looking to make some extra progress in defining your arms, this a good piece of equipment to invest in.

Ankle and wrist weights are inexpensive and can be used for a majority of the Pilates exercises. The intensity they add will benefit the advanced exerciser, so you'll see them in the *Power It Up* section. Using weights is a way to work your core while giving a boost to firming and toning your arms and legs.

Finally, both the *stability ball* and the *medicine ball* are for the experienced exerciser who wants to take his or her fitness level up a notch or two. They will greatly enhance your core stabilization skills, your coordination, and your balance. And if improving your overall flexibility is a major goal, then the stability ball will introduce you to a wonderful new strategy.

You'll want to get a good mat, preferably one that you won't slip on, that will afford you some traction when you're on your toes. And have a small pillow or a couple of towels handy for proper alignment of your head (see page 52).

For more information about where to purchase any of the equipment mentioned above, take a look at the *Resources* page in the back of this book.

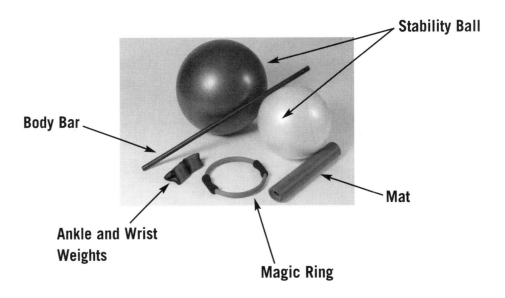

Stability Ball

Body Bar

Mat

Ankle and Wrist Weights

Magic Ring

What to Wear

Any type of clothing you're comfortable in is fine as long as it doesn't restrict movement in any direction. It's safer to avoid wearing jewelry, especially anything that hangs down or is sharp.

Pilates is generally done with bare feet because it allows for a better grip on the floor or mat. Any type of push-up is safer when there is less danger of the feet slipping. Bare feet are also highly recommended if you do any of the stability ball exercises.

Listen to Your Body

You are your own best coach. If you feel pain, stop immediately. You cannot improve by working through pain, especially joint pain. This is not the time to grit your teeth and tough it out. Find another exercise you can do right now that is challenging yet pain free. Take care of your body and it will serve you well; abuse it and it will respond accordingly. Learn to distinguish between "good hard work" and "pain," which is the harbinger of an injury. Persevere through the former, and desist with the latter.

Remember, you will have lots of opportunities to get better. And with Pilates there will be many paths to this destination.

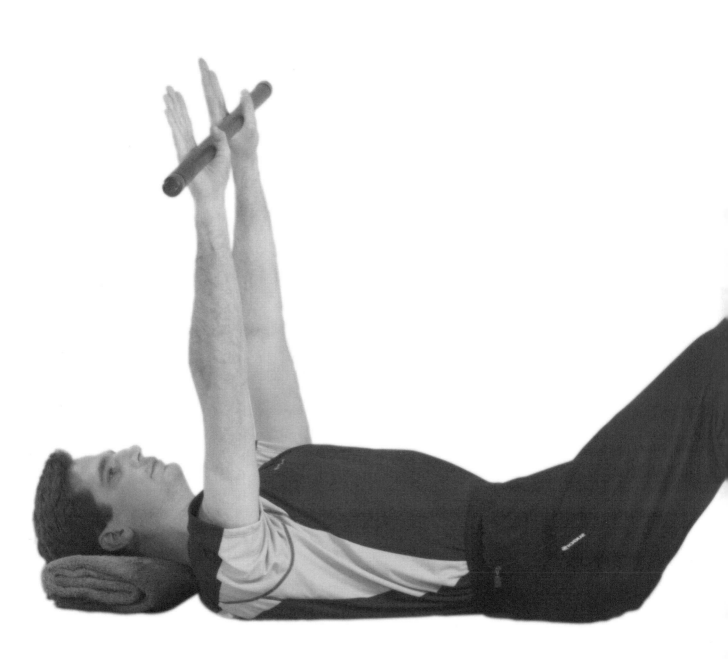

Learning the Basics

It's All About the Middle

Pilates is a full-body workout that emanates from your core. As you may recall from Chapter 2, the core consists of four muscles that comprise the abdominal wall (*rectus abdominus, internal obliques, external obliques,* and *transverse abdominus*), a muscle along your side and back (*quadratus lumborum*), and a large group of muscles that attach in varying configurations up and down and side to side along the spine from one vertebra to another (collectively known as the *erector spinae*).

Through a technique known as *stabilization* the core is engaged with every Pilates exercise.

Why *Not* Moving Is Important

Stabilization, in the context of exercise, means that one or more parts of your body are held completely still while another part of your body moves. Sound easy? In fact, it's quite difficult.

There are two types of stabilization that form the foundation of Pilates. *Pelvic stabilization* serves to exclude the muscles along the front of your thigh and groin, the *hip flexors*, from assisting with exercises geared to abdominal work.

Many people unwittingly perform crunches or curls with little or no abdominal involvement. Why? Because the body is clever; it will always want to conserve energy and reduce the effort of the task before it. Instinctively, without conscious thought, your body will try to make an exercise easier. And one way to do this is to get as many muscles as possible to participate, as when you enlist the *hip flexors* to work at the same time as the abdominals. The *hip flexors* are a bigger and stronger group of muscles. If they are taken out of the picture, then the abdominals are recruited to a much greater extent.

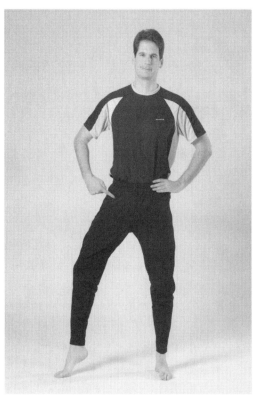

Hip flexor muscles are inhibited so abdominals get a much better workout

Another of the body's tricks to make a difficult movement easier is to use momentum, to barrel through an exercise rather than squeezing and contracting the muscles to make the action smooth and controlled. No wonder, then, that after years of traditional ab work a person may still not have "flat" abs. With pelvic stabilization, on the other hand, you create the environment for the abdominals to do the work because all the other muscles in the vicinity are prevented from assisting.

The second type of stabilization used in Pilates is *spine stabilizaton*, which anchors the upper torso. With this area immobile it is possible to *eliminate* the involvement of chest and neck muscles (*pectoralis major* and *upper trapezius*). The muscles used to stabilize the spine are the *lower trapezius* and *latissimus dorsi* (located in the middle of the back). You will be cued to "engage the lats" to keep your shoulders depressed (lowered) and your back firmly planted on the floor.

A New Look at Abdominal Training

From my years of teaching and observing students it is apparent that most people do abdominal curls incorrectly. Some by pressing their lower back down and "tucking under" their pelvis: some by pulling on their neck; some by swinging their elbows forward as they lift their head (which uses the chest muscles in lieu of abdominals); and some by sheer momentum, hurling their body forward and then allowing themselves to rock back down, letting physics do the work.

If the pelvis is stabilized, that is, if it is not tucked under as you curl up, if the hip bones do not move, if you do not pull on you head, if you do not bring your elbows forward, or develop momentum to lift off the floor—then the *only* muscle group that can lift your trunk off the floor will be your abdominals.

Laying the Groundwork

The sooner you understand and master the fundamentals, the sooner you can plunge into the Pilates repertoire.

The remainder of this chapter will fully explain, and give you the opportunity to practice, the following:

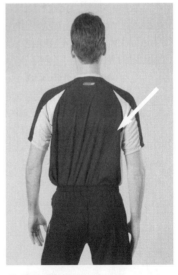

- Navel to spine
- Kegel
- Deep abdominal contraction
- Pelvic stabilization
- Engaging the lats
- Spine stabilization
- Breathing

Spine Stabilization engages the lats and lower trapezius.

Navel to Spine

Avoiding Belly Bulge

This technique allows you to access the deepest abdominal layer, the *transverse abdominus*, which is actively involved in supporting the internal organs that lie within the abdominal cavity.

As many people (especially women) grow older, they may find that their stomachs protrude, even if overall they are quite thin. The culprit is often weak abdominal musculature that does not provide adequate support for the weight and bulk of the viscera deep within the belly. Over time, the internal organs begin to push forward, expanding the belly.

Unfortunately, many of the traditional abdominal classes unwittingly train you to push the belly out.

Doing It Incorrectly

First let's feel what you should *not* do. Tuck your pelvis under so that your lower back flattens into the floor (This is the "Pelvic Tilt" described in Chapter 6). Perhaps you will tighten your buttocks or hamstring muscles. Now place one hand over your belly and lift your head off the floor. Does your stomach push into your hand? If so, you will need to take some time to unlearn this habit.

The Proper Way

Now, let's practice the right way. Inhale deeply and then exhale forcefully. As you exhale pull your navel in straight back towards your spine, which is also the direction of the floor. *Do not* tense your buttocks or hamstrings. In other words, you are *not* doing a pelvic tilt.

Correct technique will mean that you feel the *contraction*, the tightening, deep within your abdominal wall. You should feel like you are working hard, that an intensity is building up in your stomach. Avoid letting your chest sink down or your back round.

And finally, can you do all this *without* holding your breath? That's your goal. Contract the muscles as tightly as you can, hold it for a count of 5, and keep breathing all the while. You can practice this exercise in any position; seated, standing, even while reclining as you watch TV.

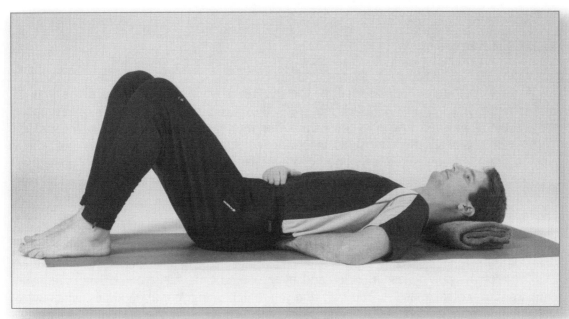

Correct: Navel to Spine *(no movement visible)*

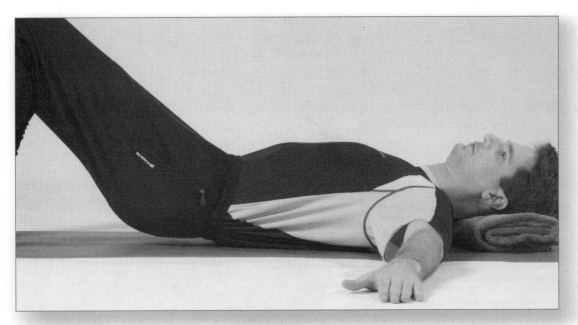

Incorrect: Pelvic Tilt *(pelvis raised, buttocks tightened)*

Kegel

What's a Kegel?

A Kegel is the *contraction* (use) of the muscle in your body that stops the flow of urine. When you perform a Kegel you "lift" the pelvic floor. There is a considerable weight being pressed into this area from the internal organs housed in the pelvis. Without strong pelvic floor muscles incontinence may result. Pregnant and post-natal woman are often prescribed a regimen of Kegel exercises to improve bladder control.

Practicing Kegels regularly helps to keep your insides strong and healthy. So feel free to do them all day—morning, noon, and night.

Doing It the Wrong Way

Contract the pelvic floor muscles and at the same time tuck your pelvis under and squeeze your buttock muscles. You may find you're tightening your abdominals (which we'll want to do shortly, but not just yet) and developing tension along the front of your hips.

Doing It Correctly

Now, let's practice the right way. Inhale deeply, and as you exhale perform a Kegel using the muscle that stops the flow of urine. Pay attention to what else is happening in your body. *Nothing* else should be happening. Relax your buttocks muscles, do not allow your hips to move or your back to press into the floor, and leave your abdominal muscles unengaged. Do this 10 times. Each time hold for a count of 5, then relax fully.

When you are clear about the isolation of the pelvic floor muscles, when you can do these 10 repetitions *and* breathe at the same time, proceed to the next basic movement, the Deep Abdominal Contraction.

Enhancing the Action

Need help with this one? Practice Kegels in conjunction with the tips in Chapter 6—but be prepared for a new awakening!

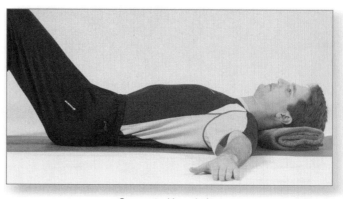

Correct: Kegel *(no movement visible)*

Deep Abdominal Contraction

The Cornerstone

When you can perform a Deep Abdominal Contraction you will be on your way to conquering pelvic stabilization, the pivotal skill required in the Pilates program.

Pull your navel in strongly *and* perform a Kegel (see page 40). The abdominals and the pelvic floor muscles will contract, but *nothing else* should occur: The pelvis does *not* tuck under and the hips do *not* move.

It's in Every Exercise

Each repetition of each Pilates exercise will require you to perform a Deep Abdominal Contraction. This might take some time to perfect, so practice these two combined movements throughout the day. Here's a trick—do it whenever you hear the telephone ring.

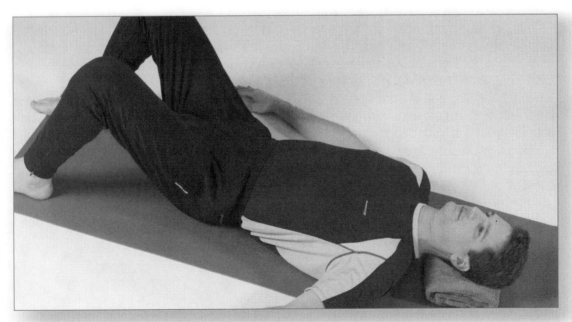

Correct: Navel to Spine with Kegel *(no movement visible)*

Pelvic Stabilization

Anatomically Speaking

The pelvic girdle is the fusion of three bones, the *ilium,* the *ischium,* and the *pubis.* When you place your hands on your hips, you're actually on the part of the pelvic girdle known as the *ilium.* If you happen to be seated upright as you read this, then you're on the part of your pelvis called the *ischium.* The *pubis* is the lower frontal portion of your pelvis. Your hip joints are the concave surfaces on either side (you can't feel these) where your thigh bones *(femurs)* connect with the pelvic girdle.

As I refer to the pelvis throughout this book keep in mind that I'm talking about the whole unit, this rather large bone, to which are attached your two leg bones on either side.

When you perform pelvic stabilization you are *cocontracting* the abdominals and back muscles to provide a stable base. When the exercise calls for you to do a Deep Abdominal Contraction it is reminding you to establish this unmoving foundation.

Anchoring Your Pelvis

Pelvic stabilization merges the two movements you've just learned, Navel to Spine and Kegel, to produce a Deep Abdominal Contraction.

Combine your muscular effort with the following visualization: create in your mind's eye the image of your pelvis as a block of heavy concrete, weighted into the floor and incapable of movement in any direction—up or down, right or left.

Practicing a Curl with Pelvic Stabilization

Lie on your back with your arms by your sides, knees bent. Do a Deep Abdominal Contraction as you lift your head off the floor. Keep your shoulders and neck down and relaxed. Do not worry about coming up very high. Just an inch or two is what we're after right now. As you curl up look toward your **right** knee. Has anything happened at your **left** hip? Has it come off the floor at all? Is there any shifting of the weight along your lower back? Your goal is *no* movement whatsoever. Use the Deep Abdominal Contraction and the image of your pelvis as a block of cement to prevent any shift from occurring.

Don't get discouraged. You likely won't be able to achieve true pelvic stabilization without many months of practice. Fortunately, in your striving you will begin to amass the benefits of Pilates, perhaps even seeing early on that your stomach is starting to flatten.

How will you know you're on the right track? Here's a hint: If an exercise feels easy, then you're *not* doing it correctly. On the other hand, if you feel a burning sensation deep within your belly, you've gotten the hang of it.

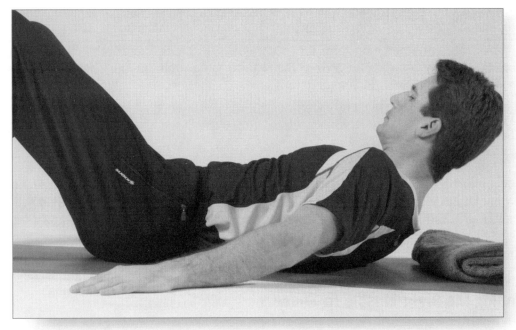

Correct: Curl up right, left side of back on the floor

Engaging the Lats

Anatomically Speaking

The "lats" (the common term for the *latissimus dorsi* muscle) originate under your armpits and form a large part of your back, from the bottom of your shoulder blades all the way down to the top of your buttocks.

The Rationale

Throughout this program you will be directed to "engage your lats" to avoid using your upper back muscles (specifically the *upper trapezius,* which raises your shoulders) and neck muscles (which can lead to spasms). The cue, "keep your shoulders down and relaxed" will call upon you to do a mild contraction of the lat muscles and *lower trapezius* to eliminate the unattractive "hunching up" of the shoulders and assist with spine stabilization (see below).

Finding the Right Muscle to Squeeze

Lift both shoulders up, and then bring them back down but actually press them down a little further. What muscle do you enlist to make your shoulders move down more? Do the action several times until you're clear where this additional pressing down movement is generated. Make a kinesthetic memory of this place so you know where to direct your attention when called upon to relax your shoulders.

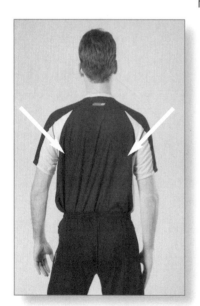

The lats

If you have a Magic Ring, lie on the floor, knees bent, and hold the ring comfortably out in front of your chest. Have your fingers long and relaxed, not gripping the ring. Direct your attention to the area at the level of your armpit along the side of your back as you lightly put pressure on the ring.

Pay attention to an important distinction: the direction of the movement is a downward one. You should *not* be pinching your shoulder blades together. Be quite certain that you avoid doing this.

Still having trouble finding the right spot? Lie on the floor with your knees bent and arms along your sides, palms down. Now reach with your fingers towards your heels as if you want to touch them. Allow your shoulder blades to move downward but be sure to avoid rounding your shoulders forward or off the floor. Put that feeling into your muscle memory bank and carry it over to your performance of the Pilates exercises.

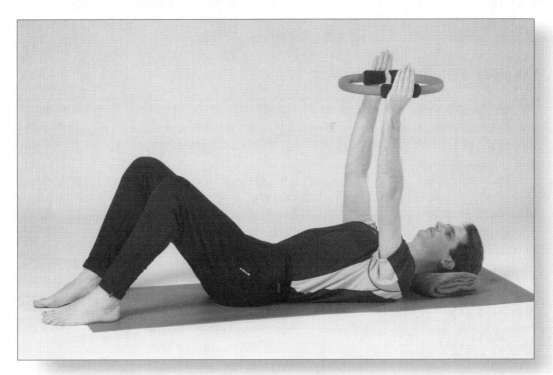

Squeezing Magic Ring

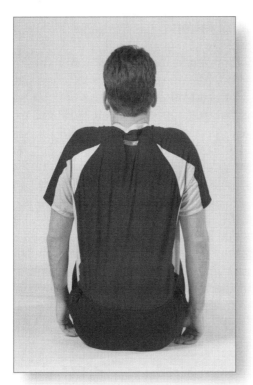

Incorrect: Shoulders hunched

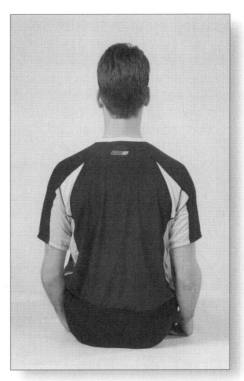

Correct: Lats engaged, shoulders pressed down

Spine Stabilization

Creating a Stable Base for Arm Work

Here's a simple movement to do while seated or standing. Lift your **right** arm overhead and reach up as high as you can. Did you bend a little to your **left** with your torso as you did this? Or did you hold your torso completely rigid so there was no movement of your rib cage?

Both strategies could be correct, but only in the latter did you perform spinal stabilization, moving your arm through space while the rest of your upper body remained immobile.

Spine stabilization is simply using the technique of Engaging the Lats (see page 44) to anchor your upper torso when you move your arms.

The Rationale

Anchoring the spine helps protect your back. It does this by recruiting more of your body's musculature, thereby decreasing the vulnerablity of individual muscles to injury.

The more of you that is actively being stabilized, the greater the ability of the exercises to achieve their targeted strengthening objectives *and* the greater safety to you when performing them.

Practicing a Pullover with Spinal Stabilization

Lie on your back with your knees bent. Hold a weight, body bar, or towel stretched out over your head (resting in the direction of the floor behind you in a comfortable spot). Now bring your arms over to your mid-chest area. Return to the starting position.

Let's add the features that transform this pullover movement into a Pilates exercise. First, bring your awareness to your lats. Now initiate the movements from this place on your back. At the same time perform pelvic stabilization, anchor your back, and lengthen your neck so your chin is slightly down. Your goal is to eliminate any bending of your chest area, any rounding of your shoulders, or any movement of your head. The *only* moving parts should be your arms. Try this and see the effect of this new focus.

Do you feel a difference? Don't you find that more effort is needed? If you're doing it correctly you are indeed working harder because you are engaging more of your body. Sounds almost like a paradox. Yet *eliminating* movement requires that muscles are recruited to contract in their isometric (non-moving) fashion, and an isometric contraction is one that quickly builds up tension in the muscle, producing a greater intensity and requiring considerable more exertion.

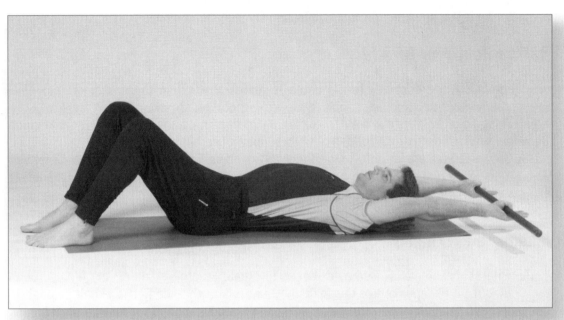

Starting Position: Arms overhead holding body bar

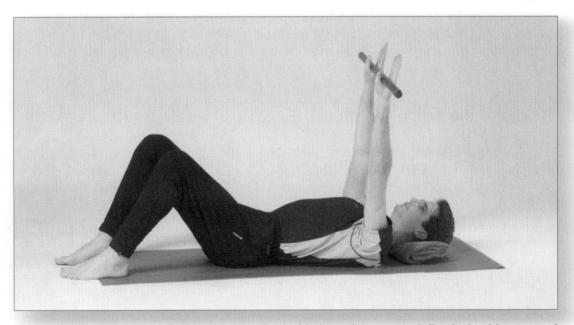

Action: Arms over to mid chest, lats engaged *(back should not move)*

Breathing

Do You Hold Your Breath?

While it sounds contradictory, Pilates is about strength without tension. So how, then, can we control and exert our muscles without tensing our body? By *using* our breath instead of *holding* our breath. We are all so geared up to make a great effort when we exercise that the natural tendency is to suspend breathing.

If you find you are unable to perform an exercise without holding your breath or without feeling great strain, use one of the Power It Down options, or choose another exercise more compatible with your present level of fitness.

Inhaling and Exhaling

In Pilates the inhale is used as a means to create length—think of air going through the body until it escapes out of the feet, the hands, and the head. The exhale is used to give energy to your movement *and* as a means to keep the body in a relaxed state.

Let's practice the correct breathing technique. Place your hands on your lower ribs. Inhale deeply through your nose and feel the air enlarge your torso. Imagine your ribs expanding like a ball. (Your ribs are not only in the front and side of your body, they totally encompass your whole torso, all the way around the back). Now exhale fully through your mouth, pushing the air out. Pay attention to where this breath is coming from. Think of the air coming from your lungs, not your belly, so that the exhalation completely expels all the air from the lungs and relaxes your ribs downward in the direction of your feet. Each time you inhale try to enlarge your rib cage even more, and each time you exhale try to compress your lungs more completely.

Enhancing the Action

You will be challenged by the paradoxical nature of the Feldenkrais-inspired Breathing sequence, presented in the Chapter 6. It will give you a new appreciation of your respiratory capabilities.

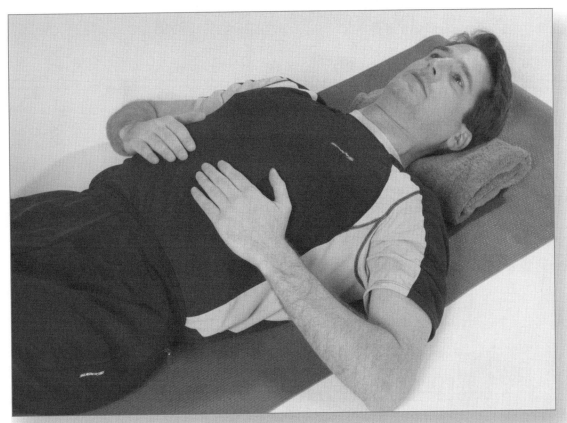

Hands on lower ribs

Form and Alignment

A "Look" with a Purpose

*E*very part of your body is attended to in Pilates, from head to toes to fingers. How you position your body not only adds to the beauty of the performance, it helps protect you from injury. No detail is too small; each has a reason routed in biomechanics, muscle recruitment, or esthetics.

Our bodies are designed to move optimally according to the structure of our joints. How and where we position ourselves allows us to exercise with the greatest range of motion within the safest possible parameters.

In paying attention to form we can control which muscles are to be used, and which are not. To achieve the Pilates "look" the right muscles must be engaged so that other muscles can relax.

In physiological terms, when we *contract* a muscle we cause it to shorten. At the same time, when a muscle is contracted it causes the *antagonist* muscle to lengthen. For example, if you were to contract your biceps, the muscle group on the front part of your upper arm, you would cause the triceps, which lie on the back of the upper arm, to be stretched out a little.

If you would like muscles that are elongated, rather than tight and bulky, you will need to faithfully and consistently adhere to the guidelines for proper technique.

This chapter will teach you the following:

- Relaxing the Neck and Shoulders
- Head Alignment
- Turning Out From the Hip
- Lengthening Out of the Sockets
- Lifting Up While Sitting
- Pointing and Flexing the Foot
- Hand and Finger Positioning

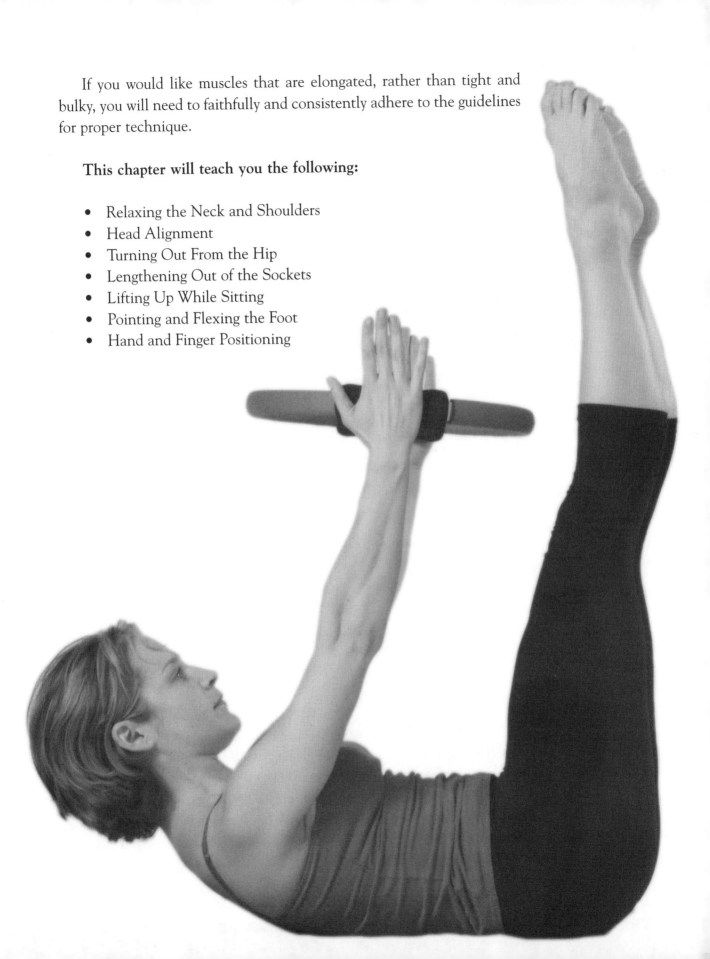

Relaxing the Neck and Shoulders

Blame It on Life's Stresses

Many people deposit their daily worries and anxieties into their neck and shoulders. The undesirable consequence may be persistent discomfort in that area, created by chronic muscle tension.

It is not uncommon for some people to approach any difficult or seemingly demanding task with a habitual "tensing" up of the shoulders and neck. What happens when a muscle is under constant impetus to contract? In addition to pain, the consequence is the decidedly non-Pilates look of an enlarged neck and hunched up shoulders.

Cues for Proper Alignment

You will receive constant reminders to pay special attention to this part of your anatomy. "Relax the shoulders," "keep your head free from tension," and "use your lats" are various cues to assist you.

Enhancement

Get acquainted with two movement patterns in Chapter 6, Shoulders Up and Down and Shoulders Together and Apart. They will make you aware of how you are holding yourself and enable you to instantly replace rigidity with relaxation.

Head Alignment

Our Natural Predilection

Our cultural predisposition is to lean forward—sometimes as a gesture of polite attentiveness, and other times because we need to see or hear better. This "forward head" position has potential ramifications down the road. Often, it is the root of eventual neck, shoulder, and even back pain. If it creates short or tight muscles it may make it impossible for you to lie down on your back without substantially arching or curving your neck.

Checking Your Head Alignment

Even if you don't experience any tightness, take a moment to pay attention to the position of your head and determine your pattern. *It is my experience that most people are unaware when they are in an unsafe neck alignment.*

Lie on your back and see if you can tell at what spot the back of your head makes contact with the floor. Chances are it's towards the top of your head, with your chin pointing upward.

Change the contact point so that it's closer to the base of your skull. This means your chin will tilt *down slightly* and you will have the feeling of a *gentle* stretch or lengthening at the back of your neck. Try using a pillow or a couple of towels for elevation and feel whether you have a sense of increased comfort.

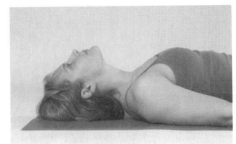

Incorrect: Chin pointing up

Where Are You Looking?

It's so ingrained in the gym mentality that I find it difficult to stop people from "looking up at the ceiling" as they lift their head off the floor. There is no value in this approach and there is a large downside—straining and bulging neck muscles.

When you lift your head up allow it to bend forward in a natural arc so your chin comes nearer to your chest and your eyes look more or less between your legs.

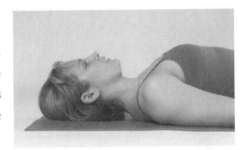

Correct: Chin tilting down

Enhancement

If you practice Holding Up Your Head in Chapter 6, you will easily be able to achieve the proper form. Your body will quickly learn these new movement patterns and you'll soon be able to lift your head up from the floor much higher, and hold it there longer with considerably less effort.

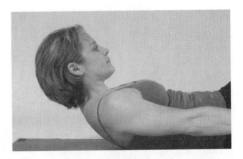

Correct: Bending forward (*no strain*)

From the Prone Position

Performing exercises when face down, such as push ups, also requires attention to neck alignment. Your goal is to keep your head aligned with your spine, as if your head is an extension of your spine (which it is). This means you neither look up nor look down. Your head should not "droop" nor should it "arch back."

Turning Out From the Hip

Pilates Stance

You will be cued to "squeeze the sides of your buttocks and backs of your upper legs" as the impetus to turn your legs out from the hip joint. Don't think of turning your feet out; initiating from the feet can cause stress to the knee joint. Allow your feet to just turn out as a natural result of the hip rotating outwards.

As is always the case with Pilates, this attention *to where* the contraction originates has important implications. Some muscles are being inhibited so others can be recruited. In this instance we are eliminating the front thigh muscles (*quadriceps*) so you don't get a "bulked up" look to your legs. At the same time we're engaging the buttocks, as well as the outer and inner thighs; the areas that most of us want lifted, toned, or sculpted.

Practicing the Movement

Lie on your back with your legs resting on the floor in an extended position. Your goal is to outwardly rotate your upper thigh bone (*femur*) to get your legs in a "turn out" position. Begin by tightening the sides of your buttock muscles (*gluteals*),

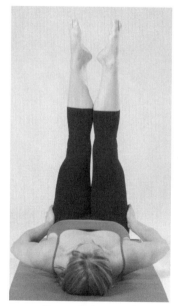
Correct: Legs raised in Pilates Stance

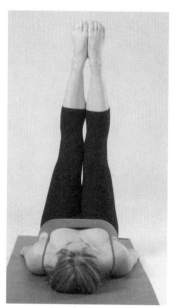
Incorrect: Legs raised, not turned out

and allow the back of your thigh muscles (*hamstrings*) and inner thigh muscles (*adductors*) to contribute. Keep your feet relaxed. *Do not* begin by turning your feet out.

Now try the Pilates Stance with both legs straight up in the air so that they form a 90 degree angle with your body (if this is uncomfortable bend your knees). Again, allow your legs to turn out from the contraction of your buttocks and upper portion of your outer and inner thighs. Remember to avoid *tensing* the front thigh muscles. Let your feet turn out in response to the rotation from your upper thighs; do not force them.

Lengthening Out of the Sockets

Our Usual Patterns

Most of our days are spent *compressing* our bodies. We're either hunched over in front of a computer, reclining as we watch TV, slumping into one hip as we stand, or slouching as we walk. Pilates reverses the toil of these everyday behaviors through its emphasis on lengthening the muscles and aligning the skeleton into efficient posture.

Throughout the Pilates program you'll be directed to "reach through your arms, hands, fingers or legs" which *decompresses* the shoulders and hip joints (often called the shoulder *sockets* and hip *sockets*) by putting more space between a bone (e.g. the *humerus*, or the *femur*) and how it sits in its respective joint. This is the antithesis and antidote to habitual jamming *into* the joints, which is the norm for most people.

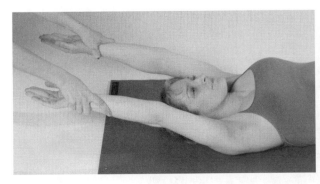

Lengthening arms out of sockets

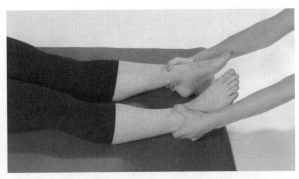

Lengthening legs out of sockets

Another cue will be to get a sense of "lengthening your waistline" by increasing the distance between the top of your hip bones and your bottom rib.

Imagery can be helpful. You might visualize a ray of light being emitted from your feet and your hands, like a burst of energy taking your arms and legs further and further away from your body. Or you can pretend someone is actually trying to pull your arms out of the shoulder socket and your legs out of the hip socket.

Go Ahead and Try It

Lie on your back with your arms overhead. Now reach through both arms and feel your ribs move upwards. Is your waistline being stretched? Do you sense your torso getting longer? Are you any taller?

Enhancing the Movement

A wonderful way to not only learn *how* to lengthen but to actually *be lengthened* is put forth in the Release exercise, Full Body Stretch, page 104.

Lifting Up While Sitting

Is This Difficult For You?

Sitting on the floor comfortably is a challenge for many of us. Chances are you lean backward a little, or your spine rounds, or perhaps your shoulders hunch up. You may feel restricted by stiff leg muscles or a tight lower back—or you may have just acquired a habit of poor sitting posture.

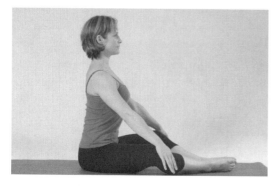

Correct: Seated, leaning slightly forward of pelvis

Tips for Improved Sitting

Sit on a chair or on the floor in a position that's as comfortable as you can make it. Where does the bottom of your pelvic bone (the *ischium*, also called the *sitting bone*) make contact? Lift your chest up, straighten your spine, and notice a shift forward on your sitting bone. Lengthen out of your waist, creating more space between your bottom rib and the top of your hip bone. Think of sitting *slightly forward* of your hips whenever you're in a seated position.

Enhancement

If you'd like to mitigate any discomfort in this posture, practice Sitting Comfortably, page 74.

Pointing and Flexing the Foot

Why Is This Important?

Proper activation and placement of the foot keeps your whole leg in good alignment, which is pivotal in preventing injury to the knees and hips. It can also help you avoid foot or toe cramping, which commonly occurs with muscle tension. And finally, it can enhance the flexibility of the foot and lower leg by stretching two areas that are frequently overworked—the calf muscles and top arch of the foot.

Don't Curl the Toes Under

When an exercise calls for you to "point your foot," do not point or curl your *toes*. Instead, see if you can create a stretch along the top of your ankle and top of your foot (instep). The toes should remain relaxed.

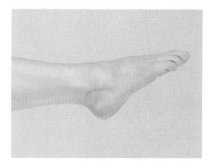

Correct: Pointed foot

Don't Flex the Toes Back

The cue to "flex your foot" should be accomplished by leading with your heel and then pulling the top of your foot closer to your shins. Sense the stretch occurring at the back of your ankle and up the back of your lower legs. Again, there is no involvement of the toes.

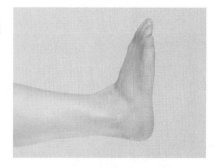

Correct: Flexed foot

Hand and Finger Positioning

You will go a long way toward keeping your entire body free of tension by relaxing and lengthening your fingers. When you hold a body bar, for example, your fingers should be off the bar and long, so that the weight of the bar is supported in your palm between your thumb and forefinger.

When your weight is supported by your hands, as in a Push-Up, keep your fingers pointing straight ahead. If you feel any stress or pain in your wrist, however, try placing your knuckles on the floor instead and see if this feels any better. If your discomfort persists, many of the exercises illus-

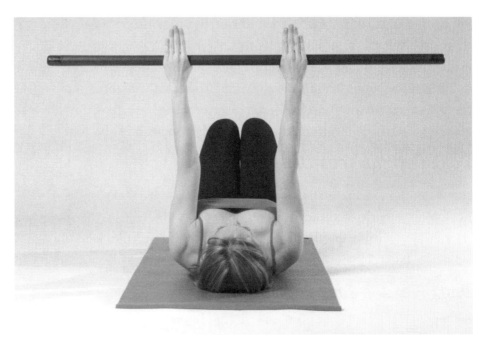

Correct: Palms support weight of body bar

trated on the hands can be performed by supporting yourself on your forearms. (See the Power It Down version of the Push-Up, page 174).

Hands should be *directly* under your shoulders for Push-Ups. Many people tend to have their hands wide apart and somewhat in front of them. You will be in better biomechanical alignment—and therefore put less stress on your shoulders, elbows and wrist—if you follow the directions above. But be prepared: if this is not your usual hand placement it will make the exercise considerably more difficult. You may not be able to bring your chest nearly as close to the floor when you bend your elbows.

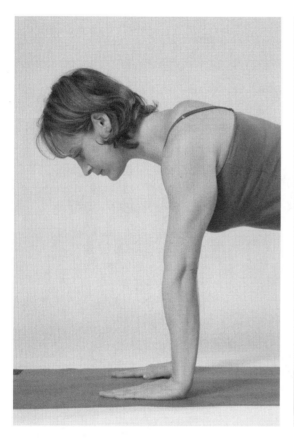

Push-Up on hands

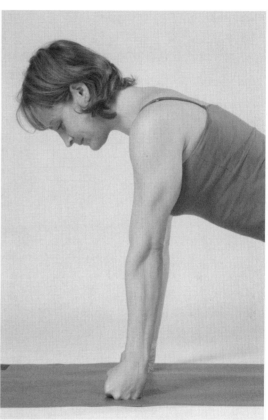

Push-Up on knuckles

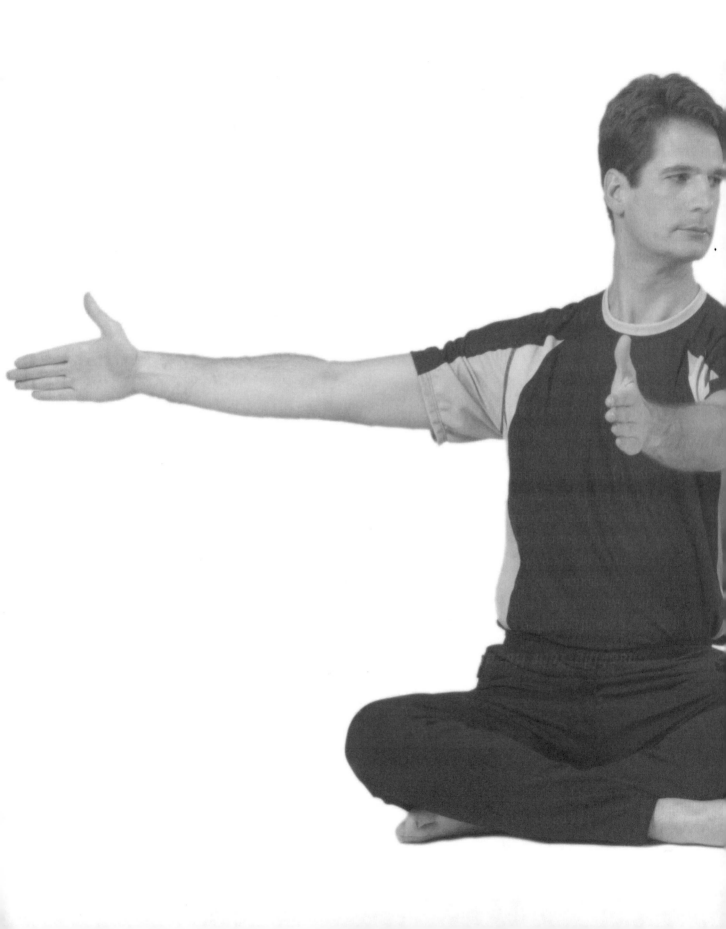

Chapter 6

The Secrets to Good Pilates Technique

A New Synthesis

Graceful, elegant, poised, flexible, strong, balanced. A combination of visual delight with physical power. Would you like to find the path that will help you acquire this type of body?

Sometimes a little ingenuity is needed, which is just what you will find in this chapter. Here you'll find ideas inspired by a method called Feldenkrais, named after its creator, Moshe Feldenkrais, who, like Joseph Pilates, developed it to cure his own debilitating condition.

Is your back always tight? Are your hamstrings too inflexible to ever straighten your knees? Do your shoulders always stay lifted, giving you a hunched look? Does it feel difficult to lift and hold your head away from the floor? Or your legs up in the air? Are you tight in your hips or inner thighs? If you would like to see improvement in any or all of these areas, then this chapter is for you.

The Power of Feldenkrais

Those who have tried Feldenkrais sing its praises. However, the technique is still largely unknown. From one end of the spectrum to the other, from the impaired to the athletic, from the movement challenged to the gifted sports professional, Feldenkrais can make a difference. All along the continuum of health, fitness, and ability, Feldenkrais is able to interject greater versatility and freedom of movement.

Feldenkrais can be described as a type of *neuromuscular* retraining that gives the brain an opportunity to learn, or relearn, ways to move with ease and comfort. When applied to the average person it can address common aches and pains or, as I'll be using it in this book, lessen musculoskeletal restrictions. Simply put, Feldenkrais increases your movement options.

Moshe Feldenkrais (1904–1984) was a man ahead of his time and only now is science beginning to catch up to his genius. Controlled research studies are revealing that Feldenkrais does indeed work, and our recently enhanced understanding of how the brain functions is beginning to elucidate *why* it works.

How Does the Magic Happen?

The "secrets" that you will learn in this chapter work because they focus on changing your normal habits. They break patterns that your body has used, probably for many years, and teach the brain to solve the movement puzzle in new ways that add greater ease, efficiency, and enjoyment. These improvements occur because additional elements of your body are called upon to participate in the action.

If your shoulder hurts, don't just look to what is happening inside the shoulder joint. The answers may lie elsewhere: your rib cage may not have adequate mobility; your shoulders blades may fail to rotate; your spine may not twist properly. You will learn to think of your body as a unified whole and begin to see how different parts of your body affect each other.

One of the key ingredients to a pain free back, for example, may be freedom of the pelvis to move in any direction. Many back specialists focus on strengthening and stretching the abdominals and the *erector spinae* (muscles of the back). The Feldenkrais Method proposes that the *entire* body is involved, and does not limit itself to the specific part or parts of the body that are suffering. One of the key ingredients to a pain free back, for example, may be freedom of the pelvis to move in any direction. It is no surprise then, with the majority of Americans likely to become afflicted with back pain at some point in their lives, that most of the people I have seen in my work over the years have limited pelvic movement.

An Unbeatable Combination

Pilates and Feldenkrais have in common their focus on the pelvis. But in other ways, Pilates and Feldenkrais are the antithesis of one another. Developing coordinated muscular strength and awareness to *prevent* movement through stabilization is the goal of the former, and acquiring new options to *enable more* movement is the achievement of the latter. I believe that pairing them can facilitate powerful changes in your body.

Because the focus of this book is Pilates, I have truncated the sequences in this chapter so they last a few moments. Generally, a full Feldenkrais lesson is about forty-five minutes long.

Contained in this chapter are powerful mini-processes from which you can derive a noticeable difference in just a short time. They cannot, however, deliver the benefit of a full Feldenkrais experience. We each have our own internal body mysteries that propel us to move in certain ways. The sequences I've chosen to put on the page may not be sufficient to unravel your somatic secrets. If you experience no change, or if you'd like to achieve greater progress, take a look at Chapter 11: *Strategies for Improving*.

The possibilities for learning how to move better are infinite. Any additional time you can spare to learn more about Feldenkrais will add to your life immeasurably. You will find yourself turning to this method again and again as a way to enhance just about any endeavor or pursuit you undertake.

Your Mantra for Discovering New Possibilities

As you explore the movements in this chapter, continually remind yourself of the following:

- There should be no pain; stop immediately if feel any pain.
- Start with simply imagining yourself following the instructions.
- Next, do a tiny movement such that a person looking at you could not even see anything occurring.
- Gradually, with no force or effort involved, allow the range of motion to increase until you achieve a comfortable, non-straining, range of motion.
- You never need to attain your possible end point or maximum stretch. Stop at some point in the middle of your ability, not where you could be if you really pushed yourself.
- Do not try to match the models in the photos. Your body may move differently, or to a lesser or greater degree.
- Go slow, the slower the better.
- Perform each movement in the easiest, simplest, least straining way you know how.
- Scan your body for any unnecessary tension and attempt to let go of it.
- Pay attention to your breathing. Do not hold your breath. Discover for yourself whether exhaling or inhaling helps with each step along the way.

Other key points to bear in mind:

- Do at least the fewest number of repetitions listed for each series—but always feel free to do more.
- Take a rest between *each* direction for a brief moment—and you can rest more often if you wish.
- When you rest you can choose to return to the starting position, you can lie down on your back, or you can find another comfortable position.
- It bears repeating again: stop if you feel pain. Simply do the entire sequence in your imagination. As unbelievable as it sounds, this will be enough to make noticeable improvements.

Do you think your muscles are just too tight or stiff to attain the Pilates body? Be prepared to start bending, stretching, and moving in ways you thought were utterly impossible.

Here is an overview of what you will learn in this chapter:

- Rotation
- Holding the Head Up
- Pelvic Tilt
- Head Drop Back
- Sitting Comfortably
- Kegel
- Shoulders Up and Down
- Arms Lying Straight Overhead
- Shoulders Together and Apart
- Hamstring Flexibility
- Inner Thigh Flexibility
- Hip Flexor Flexibility
- Holding the Legs Up
- Preparing for Back Work I
- Preparing for Back Work II
- Breathing
- Rolling

Rotation

PURPOSE

Turning takes a supple spine, but it also requires involving your whole body to move in a coordinated way. Creating a fully mobile spine is one of the goals embedded in the Pilates method and with the following Feldenkrais-influenced series of movements you will immediately sense a new freedom and perhaps even awe of your body's power to so easily improve.

PILATES EXERCISES

This enhancement will help with all Pilates exercises that require you to rotate your spine: Seated Twist, Bicycle, Scissors.

ACTION

Sit with your legs apart comfortably or in a cross-legged position. Bring your arms to the halfway point between straight out in front and straight out to the side. Twist your torso to the **right**, and then to the **left**. Notice how far you turn in each direction.

REPETITIONS

Do each movement slowly, easily, without trying too hard, 4 times (only a very few repetitions are needed for this one).

ENHANCING THE ACTION

1. Perform the action above. Try to maintain the distance between your arms as you twist to the **right**. Just do what's easy. Then twist to the **left**. Listen to your body. How far can you easily twist? Do you immediately tense your shoulders? Do you hold your breath?
2. This time, as you twist your torso to the **right**, turn your head to look to the **left**, and as you twist to the **left**, turn and look to the **right**.
3. Now, turn your *body* to the **right** and your *head* to the **left**, but this time take your eyes to the **right**. Then reverse it—turn your body to the **left** and your head to the **right** but turn your *eyes* to look to the **left**.
4. Do the initial movement. Can you turn farther now?

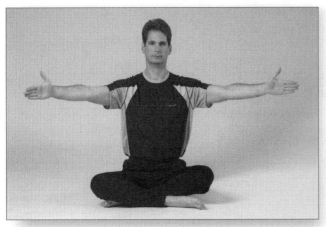

Action: Arms extended

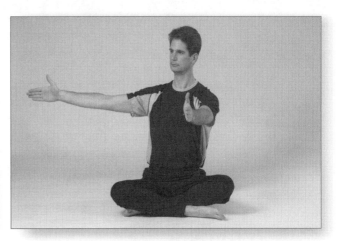

Action: Torso twist right

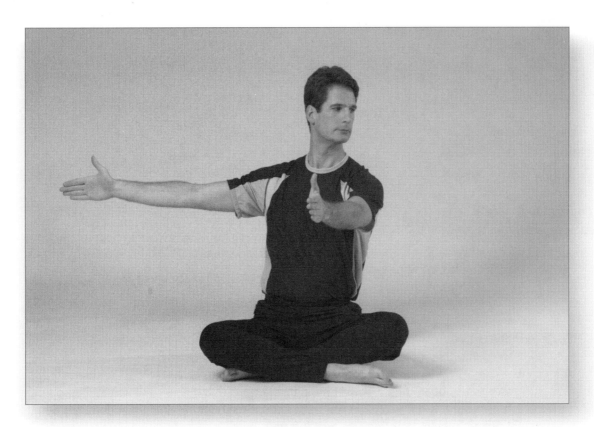

Enhancement No. 2: Torso twist right, head turn left

Holding the Head Up

PURPOSE

An integral part of the Pilates repertoire is the ability to lift the head off the floor and keep it lifted for an extended period of time. It would be natural to assume that strong neck muscles need to be developed. Surprisingly, your ability to accomplish this maneuver relies on good bodily "organization" rather than muscle strength. For example, your chest must soften and your ribs must move downward to make this move easy. If you find that keeping your head lifted without support for more than a second or two is impossible for you, this sequence will change that immediately.

PILATES EXERCISES

Breathing to 100, Single Leg Stretch, Straight Leg Stretch, Legs Lower and Lift, Crisscross, Scissors, Double Leg Extension, Teaser—and all of the abdominal exercises that require you to lift and then lower your head.

ACTION

Lie on your back with your knees bent. Lift your head off the floor. Imagine you were going to hold it up for an hour. Could you?

REPETITIONS

With the least amount of effort possible, do each movement 4 to 6 times.

ENHANCING THE ACTION

1.   Lie on your back with your knees bent and your feet flat on the floor. Lift your head up and notice which way you   eyes move. Do they look forward, or move up, or even m o v e down?

2.   Lift your head and try to look behind you, not up to the ceiling, but as if you're trying to see the wall through the back of your head.

3.   Place both feet on the floor. Now lift your heels up. What happens at your lower back? Accentuate this movement of your back.

4.   This time lift your toes up. What happens at your lower back? Does it come a little closer to the floor? Allow that to happen even more.

5.   Lift both feet off the floor, and bring your knees to your chest. Bring your hands behind your head, elbows pointing forward. Lift your head up and bring your knees a little bit toward your elbows and your elbows a little bit toward your knees. Place your head back down to rest completely between each repetition.

6.   Lift your head up and bring your knees *away* a little bit from your elbows and your elbows away from your knees. Your head should return to rest on the floor after each effort.

7.   Put your feet back down on the ground. Place your hands on your bottom ribs. Press the ribs down gently toward your feet (be sure you are not pressing toward the floor).

8.   Move your hands to your breastbone. Again, press down gently towards your feet.

9.   Place one hand on a spot on your breastbone. Think of lifting your head up from this spot.

10.   Now come back to the original test movement. Your knees should be bent so your feet are on the floor. Just lift your head. Has it become lighter?

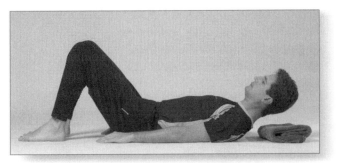

Action: Feet flat, head up

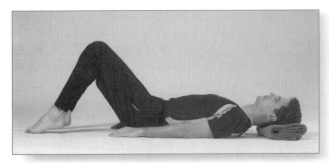

Enhancement No. 3: Heels up

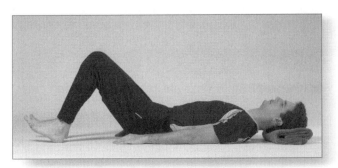

Enhancement No. 4: Toes up

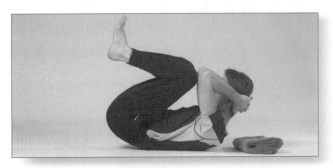

Enhancement No. 5: Knees to chest

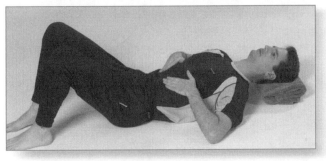

Enhancement No. 7: Rib press

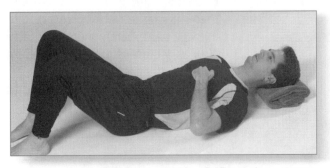

Enhancement No. 8: Breastbone press

Pelvic Tilt

PURPOSE

The ability to direct or inhibit the movements of the pelvis—forward and back, side to side, and circling—is at the core of most of the Pilates repertoire.

PILATES EXERCISE

Roll Down, Buttocks Squeezes, Cat Stretch.

PURPOSE

Tuck your pelvis under so that your lower back begins to press against the floor. Reverse the movement so that you create a hollow space between your lower back and the floor. Make the movement very small, so small that if a person was looking at you they would have difficulty seeing that you are doing anything at all. Get a sense of how clear this is for you right now.

REPETITIONS

Perform each and every movement in a pain-free, comfortable zone, with the least amount of effort, 8 to 10 times.

ENHANCING THE ACTION

1. Tuck your pelvis under gently, just a little, so that your lower back begins to press against the floor. Now reverse the movement so that you create a hollow space between your lower back and the floor.
2. Stop the movement of the pelvis. Turn your head a little to the **right**, and then a little to the **left**.
3. Combine the Pelvic Tilt movements with the turn of the head to the **right** and **left**.
4. Do the tilting at one speed while moving your head at another speed. This may seem impossible, but give it a try.
5. Stop what you've been doing and rest a moment.
6. Place the soles of your feet together. Lift your **right** hip up so you roll to the left, and then lift your **left** hip up so you roll to the **right**. Remember, begin with a microscopic movement, barely more than doing nothing at all.
7. Now as you lift your **right** hip and roll a little to the **left**, turn your head to the **left**, and return to the center.
8. This time lift your **left** hip, roll to the **right**, turn your head to the **right,** and again to the center.

9. We'll reverse it now. Lift your **right** hip and roll to the **left**, and turn your head to the **right.**
10. Next, lift your **left** hip and roll to the **right** while turning your head to the **left**.
11. Sit up and place the soles of your feet together. In this seated position, lift your **right** hip up, and then your **left** hip.
12. Still seated, hang your head way back so your chin comes away from your chest, and do a Pelvic Tilt forward and back a couple of times. (If it is difficult to bring the head back, see Drop Head Back).
13. Lie down again and do the initial Pelvic Tilt movement. Do you feel a difference from when you began to do it just a few moments ago?

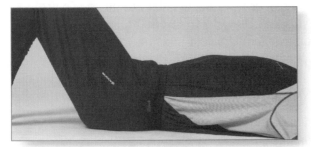

Action: Lower back flat

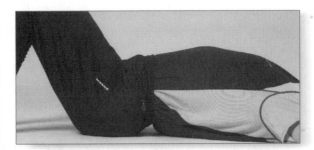

Action: Lower back arched

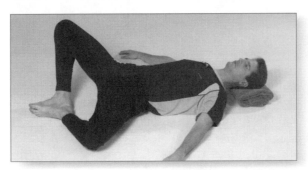

Enhancement No. 6: Hip rolling

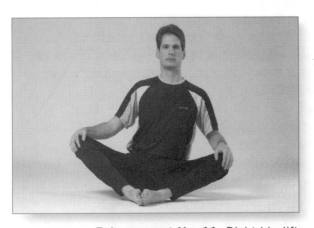

Enhancement No. 11: Right hip lift

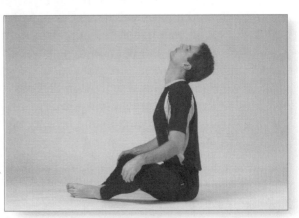

Enhancement No. 12: Head back

Head Drop Back

PURPOSE

We often hold our heads with great rigidity. Over time, this can lead to the loss of full movement potential and contribute to chronic neck and shoulder pain.

PILATES EXERCISES

Cat Stretch, Back Arch (ball).

ACTION

In a seated position (on a chair or on the floor) drop your head back as far as you can so your chin moves away from your chest. Take care of yourself. Don't try to "work through" any pain. Stay in a very small range of motion. Use micromovements, or just imagine yourself doing it. Remember to keep your hands positioned on your face. Do not try to emulate the model, as his neck bends quite far back.

REPETITIONS

Do each step 8 to 10 times, slowly, barely moving at all. Then do 8 to 10 repetitions, gradually increasing the range of motion. If you feel any pain stop immediately, and do it in your imagination.

ENHANCING THE ACTION

1. Cup your chin with both hands. The heel of your hand should support your chin and your fingers should be on your cheeks. Start by moving your head **up** 1 inch (yes, just 1 inch), and then **down** 1 inch. *Gradually* increase the distance you move your head **up** and **down** as you continue.
2. Still holding your chin, move your head **up** and look **up** with your eyes as far as you can. Then lower your chin with your eyes also looking down.
3. Still holding your chin, move your head **up** and look **down**. Then reverse the action. As you move your head **down**, look **up** and try to see the top of your head.
4. With your hands still cupping your chin, turn your head slightly to the **right.** Lift your head **up** and **down** in this new position. Gradually increase the range of motion. Feel movement occurring at your back, that your back is bending and arching. Do the same with your head turned 45 degrees to the **left**.
5. Bring your arms down. Do a Pelvic Tilt, forward and backward, a few times.
6. Then cup your chin and lift your head up as you do a Pelvic Tilt forward (so your back arches), and backward (so your back rounds).
7. Repeat the original movement. Do you feel a difference?

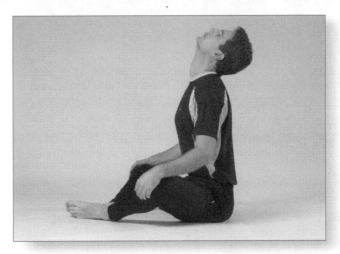

Action: Head back

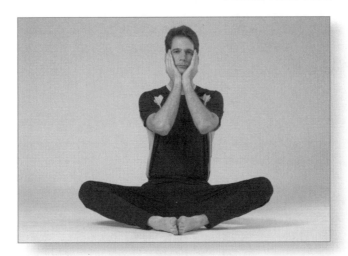

Enhancement No. 1: Chin cup

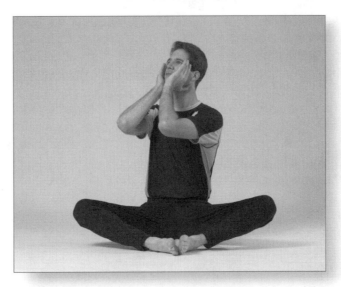

Enhancement No. 4: Chin cup with head turn right

Sitting Comfortably

PURPOSE

Many of us spend a considerable portion of our days perched on a chair or snuggled into a couch. Orthopedists and physical therapists have known for years that when we are seated we are contributing *more* stress to our backs than if we were in any other position.

PILATES EXERCISES

Spine Stretch, Seated Twist, Roll Down.

ACTION

Sit in a diamond shape position, the soles of your feet together or nearly together, with your feet a little distance away from you. You may, instead, sit in a cross-legged position. How comfortable are you as you sit?

REPETITIONS

Do each movement slowly, easily, and without forcing. Repeat 10 times imperceptibly, and 10 times progressively increasing the range of the action.

ENHANCING THE ACTION

1. Sit in a diamond shape. Hold your **right** ankle (or somewhere at the lower leg) with your **right** hand, and your **left** ankle with your **left** hand. Your thumbs should be together with the rest of your fingers.
2. Lift your **right** leg up a few inches, and then place it down. Continue to lift and lower for the recommended repetitions.
3. Now lift your **left** leg up a few inches, and then place it down for several repetitions.
4. Still holding onto your ankles, slide both feet a little bit away from you, and then slide them back in. Allow your back to round as your feet move away, and then focus on straightening your back as your feet come back in towards your body.
5. This time see if you can hold lower down your lower leg, or holding your foot if you can. Lift your **right** leg **up** and **down**. Complete the repetitions, and then repeat the action with your **left** leg.
6. Still holding onto your feet, slide both feet away from you, and then back in toward you. Augment the rounding of your back as your feet slide away, as well as the erectness of your back as your feet slide back in.
7. Sit as you did initially. Are you more comfortable now?

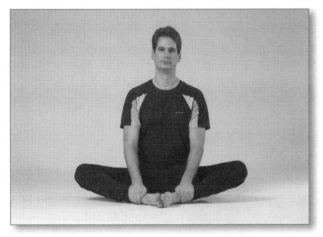

Action: Holding ankles

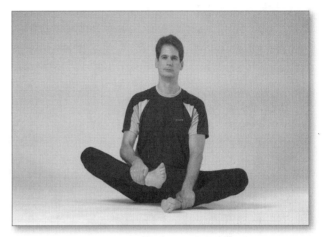

Enhancement No. 2: Right leg lift

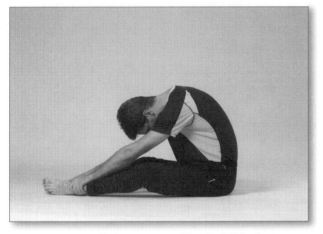

Enhancement No. 6: Slide feet away

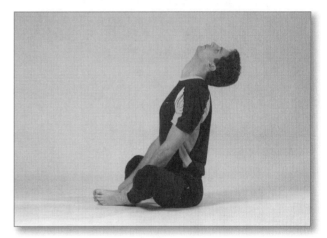

Enhancement No. 6: Pull feet back

Kegel

PURPOSE

A Kegel enables you to access the muscles of your pelvic floor. The pelvic floor can be thought of as the "basement" of your torso and so receives the weight of everything above it. Without sufficient muscle tone in your pelvic floor, incontinence may occur, especially as you get older.

PILATES EXERCISES

Every one.

ACTION

Lie on your back. Contract your pelvic floor muscles. This is what you would do if you were to stop the flow of urine. (Someone observing would not see any movement at all.) Do not tighten your stomach, squeeze your buttocks, or press your chest down. This is an internal contraction only. Is this easy to do? Can you perform it smoothly?

REPETITIONS

Do each movement slowly, easily, without forcing, about 8 to 10 times.

ENHANCING THE ACTION

1. Contract the pelvic floor so that the contraction starts in the front (from your pubic bone) and moves to the back (towards your buttocks). Don't worry if you feel you cannot do it very well in the beginning. Just try. Go slowly, easily, and don't hold your breath.
2. Contract the pelvic floor moving from back to front (the reverse of what you just did).
3. Do a Pelvic Tilt. Press your lower back down, and then reverse the movement, allowing your lower back to arch a little away from the floor.
4. As you do a Kegel, press your lower back down.
5. Keep doing the Kegel, pressing your lower back down, and start allowing your chest to participate. Make the movement bigger so that your chest starts to flatten.
6. Switch to doing a Kegel as you arch your lower back so your chest pushes forward. Start very small, and gradually increase the range of motion.
7. Squeeze just your **right** buttock as you do a Kegel. Then squeeze just the **left** buttock. Then squeeze both together.
8. Finally, *inhale* as you do a Kegel, so your stomach enlarges, then *exhale* and relax. Then *exhale* as you do a Kegel, and relax the contraction as you inhale.
9. Try the original movement again. Does it seem much clearer to you now?

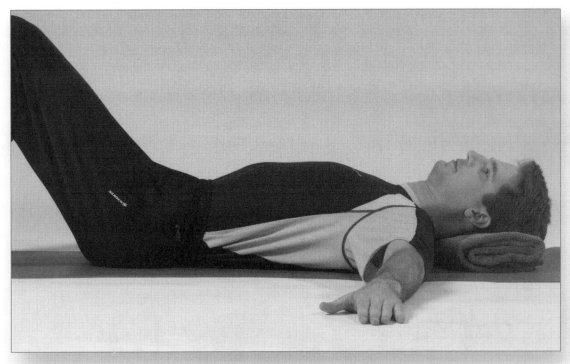

Action: Pelvic floor contraction *(no movement visible)*

Shoulders Up and Down

PURPOSE

Do you ever experience tightness or pain in your shoulders or neck? If so, it may be the result of tensing your shoulders every time you do something that requires concentration or force. With practice, it's possible to break this habit; it's part of what achieving the Pilates "look" is all about.

PILATES EXERCISES

This enhancement will help with almost the entire repertoire.

ACTION

While seated or standing (on the floor or in a chair) bring your shoulder blades **up** and **down**. How does it feel? Do they move smoothly? How far are they moving?

REPETITIONS

Slowly, easily, without strain, do about 10 imaginary or micromovements, and then 10 gradually extending your range of motion.

ENHANCING THE ACTION

1. Bring your head **up** and **down** slowly, so that your chin moves away from your chest and then toward your chest. Go slow and keep the movement very small. Do not attempt to emulate the range of movement of the model.
2. Now lift both shoulders **up** as you lift your head **up**, and let both shoulders come back **down** as you lower your head and look **down**.
3. This time as you lift your shoulders blades **up**, bring your head **down**, and as you lower your shoulder blades, lift your head **up**.
4. Next do some Pelvic Tilts so that your lower back rounds, and then arches.
5. Combine the movement of your pelvis *forward* (the back rounds) with *lifting* your shoulder blades, and the movement of your pelvis *backward* (the back arches) with *lowering* the shoulders.
6. Reverse the pattern by moving your pelvis *backward* as you *lift* your shoulders, and moving your pelvis *forward* when *lowering* your shoulders.
7. Stop everything. Simply turn your head to the **right** and **left** a few times.
8. Continue by lifting your shoulders blades as you turn your head to the **right** and **left**.
9. Keep lifting and lowering your shoulders slowly, but have a different, perhaps faster rhythm of turning your head, so the two are not "in sync."

10. Lift your **left** shoulder **up** and bend your body to the **right**; you should be doing a side bend at your waist. Then lift your **right** shoulder up and bend to the **left**.

11. Stop everything. Perform the original movement. Do you feel a new gliding ability of your shoulder blades?

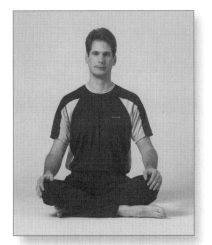

Action: Starting position

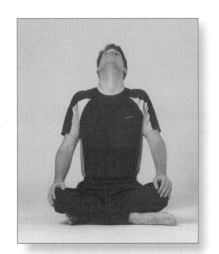

Enhancement No. 2:
Shoulders up, head up

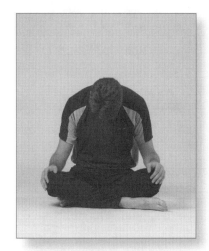

Enhancement No. 2:
Shoulders down, head down

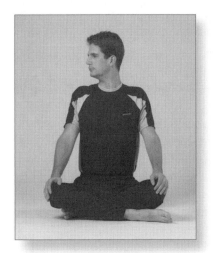

Enhancement No. 8:
Shoulders up, head turn right

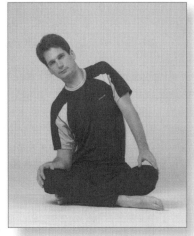

Enhancement No. 10:
Side bend right

Arms Lying Straight Overhead

PURPOSE

The beautiful arms that evolve from Pilates start with the ability to straighten the elbows completely. This extension can be difficult for many people, especially when lying on their back, arms resting overhead and resting flat on the floor behind. It may, in fact, seem impossible to make contact with the floor in this way; perhaps only your fingertips may touch at the moment. You may also notice a marked difference in the ability of one arm to reach the floor compared to the other.

PILATES EXERCISES

Roll Up, Teaser I, Full Body Stretch.

ACTION

Lie on your back. Your legs should be long on the floor. Bring both arms over your head in the direction of the floor.

REPETITIONS

Keep everything nice and easy as you do each instruction 10 times.

ENHANCING THE ACTION

1. Bring both arms overhead. Note how they are resting. Is there a difference between your **right** arm and your **left** arm? Is one arm straighter, or closer to your ear, than the other?
2. Bring your arms down by your sides. Flex your **right** foot, bringing your toes toward your shin.
3. Bring your **right** arm overhead. Reach through your **right** arm allowing your palm to turn as you perform the reaching.
4. Reach through your **right** arm as you flex your **right** foot.
5. Bring both arms overhead. Bend your **right** knee so your **right** foot is standing. Press into your **right** foot to lift your **right** hip off the floor slightly, and then lower it down.
6. Gradually increase the lift so your hip rolls to the **left**.
7. Do steps 4-6 on the other side.
8. Try the original movement with your legs long and your arms over your head. Do you feel your arms are a bit straighter now?

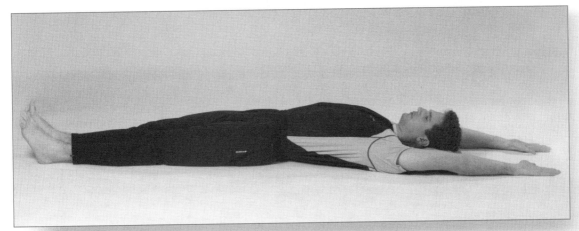

Action: Arms overhead

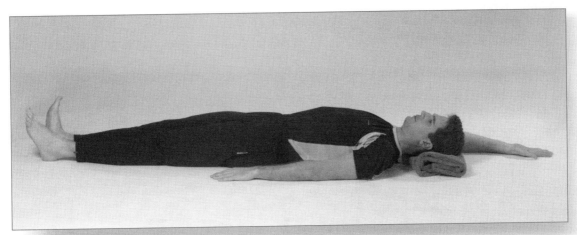

Enhancement No. 3: Right arm overhead

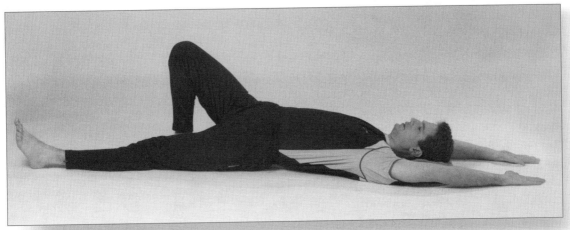

Enhancement No. 5: Right leg standing

Shoulders Together and Apart

PURPOSE

Pretend that someone has placed a pencil between your shoulder blades and you want to squeeze that pencil. How would you move? Now allow your chest to sink in and round your shoulders forward. This would be the normal position for many of us as we sit in front of a computer or at our desks. Clearly, the positioning of the shoulder blades is central to attaining proper upper body posture.

PILATES EXERCISES

This enhancement will help with Push-Ups, Push-Up Hold, and Leg Pull Front.

ACTION

While seated or standing, bring your shoulder blades together, then move them apart. Is this easy to do? Do your shoulder blades move a lot?

REPETITIONS

Gently and easily, without any big movements, do about 8 to 10 of each. You never need to go to the limit of your ability. The sequence works better if you stay small and go slow.

ENHANCING THE ACTION

1. Lie on your **left** side and lift your **right** arm up until it is parallel to the floor. With your arm in this position, reach forward so that your arm comes a little out of its socket, and then back.
2. Rotate your arm inward (your little finger lifts) as you reach forward.
3. Next rotate your arm outward (your palm turns up) as you reach forward.
4. Bring your **right** arm up so it is perpendicular to the floor. In this position, reach up. Allow your arm to rotate as you do this.
5. Watch your hand as you bring your arm up in an arc away from the floor and to the back as far as you can.
6. Repeat steps 1-5 lying on your right side.
7. Then do the original movement of the shoulder blades coming together and apart. Do you feel a difference?

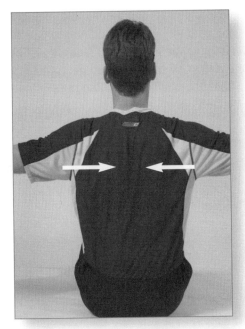

Action: Shoulder blades together

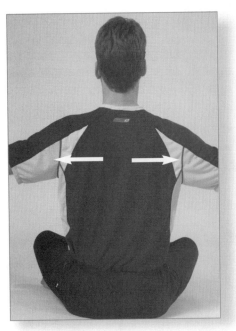

Action: Shoulder blades apart

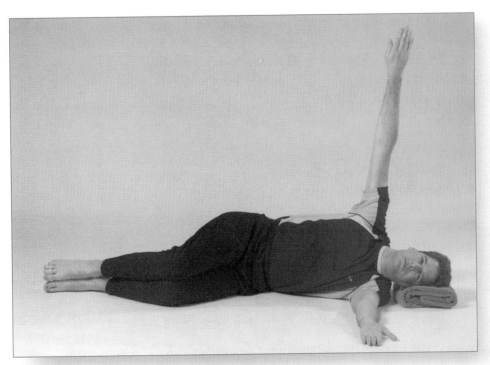

Enhancement No. 4: Right arm reach with rotation

Hamstring Flexibility

PURPOSE

Genetics play a large role in determining how flexible we are. Some of us can bend over and touch our toes while others believe that never the twain shall meet. Fortunately, with improved hamstring flexibility, every exercise will become more accessible and more possible.

PILATES EXERCISES

Straight Leg Stretch, 90/90, Legs Lower and Lift, Scissors, Jackknife, Spine Stretch, Seated Twist.

ACTION

Lie on your back. Bring your **right** leg straight up, pull it toward you, and feel the stretch in your hamstrings (the back of your thigh). Then do the same with your **left** leg. How does it feel? How far in does each leg come? (Your other leg can be long or you can keep your knee bent so the sole of your foot is on the floor)

REPETITIONS

Do each step about 10 times, beginning, as always, with an imaginary action, building to a barely perceptible movement, and then increasing from there. Do not make the biggest possible movement you can; keep it *very small, light, and without strain.*

ENHANCING THE ACTION

1. Perform Pelvic Tilts, gently and easily, pressing your lower back down just a small amount, and then arching so your lower back comes slightly off the floor. (See Pelvic Tilt).
2. Continue with the Pelvic Tilt. As you press your back down bring your chin **down**. As your back lifts from the floor bring your chin **up**.
3. Reverse the chin movement as you do the Pelvic Tilt. As you press your back **down** bring your chin **up**, and vice versa.
4. Place your hands on your upper sternum (breastbone) and slide it gently toward your feet. Move your hands 1 inch lower, and slide it down again. Continue to move your hands lower as you press on your sternum. (Be sure you are pressing in the direction of your feet and not toward the floor).
5. Now put both hands on your ribs and gently slide them in a downward motion toward your feet.
6. Let's come back to the initial stretch again. Is there an improvement?

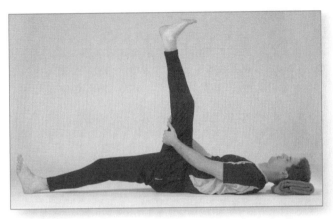

Action: Right leg up

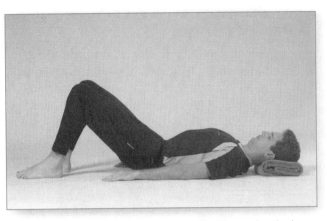

Enhancement No. 2: Chin down, back down

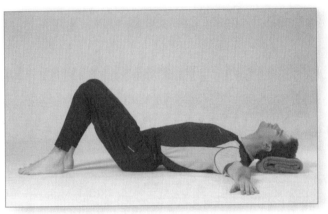

Enhancement No. 2: Chin up, back arched

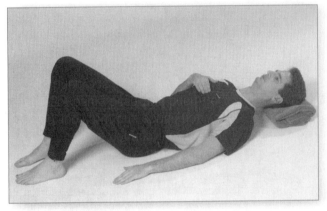

Enhancement No. 4: Breastbone press down

Inner Thigh Flexibility

PURPOSE

If you aspire to increase the flexibility of your inner thigh muscles, this Feldenkrais-based pattern can help. With an enhanced ability to spread your legs apart (the straddle position) your exercise execution will not only be more visually pleasing, but it will also give your muscles more of a workout as they contract through a greater range of motion.

PILATES EXERCISES

Inner Thigh, Pilates First, Seated Twist, Spine Stretch.

ACTION

Sit with your legs spread comfortably. Place both hands in front of you. Do not round your back. Note how far apart your legs are and how far forward you can bend.

REPETITIONS

Do each pattern 10 times microscopically, and then 10 times with greater range. Begin *very small*, and increase from there. You never need to go to your maximum range.

ENHANCING THE ACTION

1. Lie on your back. Place the outside of your **right** foot on your left thigh (so the right knee will be turned out), and bring both legs into your chest. Lift your chin, and then lower your chin. Keep your head on the floor as you do this.
2. Gradually increase the range so that when you lift your chin more of the top of your head is on the floor. (Be sure to start slowly, gradually, and stay in a pain-free range. Take care not to hurt your neck or back.)
3. As you lift your chin allow your lower back to raise off the floor.
4. Change legs, placing the outside of your **left** foot on your **right** thigh. Lift your chin and then lower it, keeping your head on the floor.
5. Note what happens in your lower back. Allow your back to arch a little away from the floor.
6. Sit with your legs spread apart a comfortable distance. Your knees can be bent or not. Place your hands in back of you. Squeeze your shoulder blades together, and then lift your chest up. Do this twice.
7. Still in the seated position, bring your shoulder blades together, lift your chest up, push your stomach forward, and drop your head back. (If this is difficult, see Head Drop Back, page 72). Bring your head back to the starting position. Do this about 5 times, dropping your head only as far as is comfortable. A very small range of motion is fine.

8. Still in the same position, bring your shoulder blades together, lift your chest, push your stomach forward and drop your head back. Hold it there and push your pelvis forward so that you create more of an arch in your lower back.

9. Sit in the initial position again with your legs spread apart. Has there been an improvement?

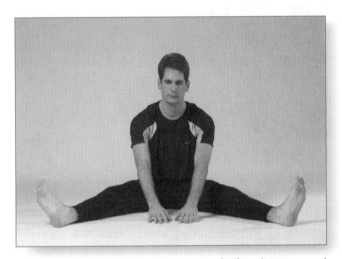

Action: Legs spread

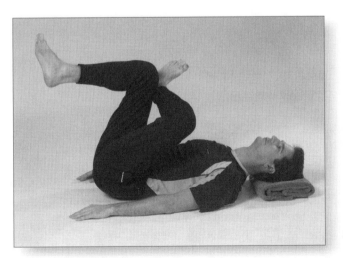

Enhancement No. 4: Left foot on right thigh

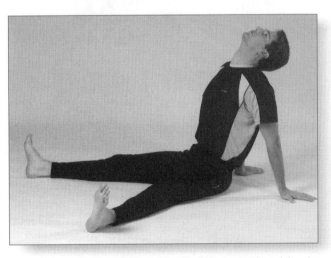

Enhancement No. 7: Chest up, head back

Hip Flexor Flexibility

To mirror the "lengthened" look of a toned Pilates leg you need sufficient *elasticity* (flexibility) of the muscles that cross the front of your hip joint. Additionally, if these muscles are tight it can, over time, lead to chronic back discomfort.

PILATES EXERCISES

Quad Stretch, Rocking; also the ability to keep the opposing leg straight in Single Leg Stretch and Straight Leg Stretch.

ACTION

Lie on your back with both knees bent, feet flat on the floor and spread far apart (more than hip distance apart). Move your **right** knee in toward the middle, keeping your **left** knee where it is. Just do what's *very* easy; do not force your knee down. Do the same with your **left** knee. How much movement is available to you?

REPETITIONS

Start *very slow and small,* using 10 barely perceptible movements and 10 with a greater range of motion.

ENHANCING THE ACTION

1. Lie on your back with knees bent, feet flat on the floor and spread far apart (more than hip distance apart).
2. Starting with just 1 inch of movement, bring your **right** knee down toward the middle without moving your **left** leg. Your **left** knee should stay pointing up. Return to starting position.
3. Bring your **right** knee down as you turn your head to the **left**. Then come back to the center.
4. This time bring your **right** knee down as you turn your head to the **right**.
5. Switch legs. Do steps 2-4 on the other leg.
6. Place both feet on the floor. Straighten your **right** leg and bring it toward you holding onto it with both hands. Keep your head on the floor and bring your eyes up as though to look behind you, and then return your eyes to the starting position. Your head should remain on the floor.
7. Still holding your **right** leg, lift your chin up slightly and then return to its starting place. The back of your head should stay on the floor.
8. Switch legs and repeat steps 6 and 7 with your **left** leg.
9. With both feet on the floor, do a Pelvic Tilt, forward and backward, 5 times or so.

10. This time bring your **right** knee down toward the middle as you arch your back a little off the floor.
11. Do the same with your **left** knee.
12. Perform the initial movement again. Does your knee come closer to the floor now?

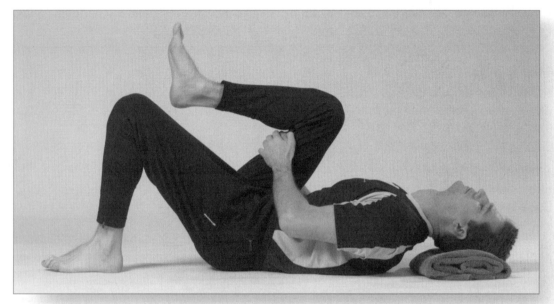

Enhancement No. 7: Right leg to chest, chin up

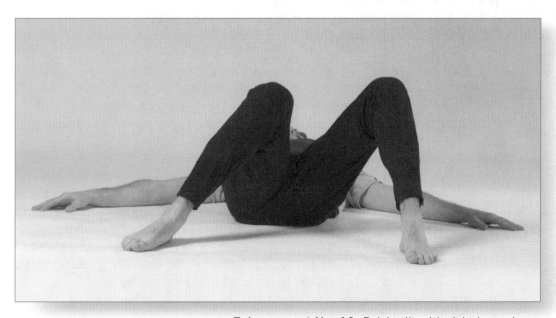

Enhancement No. 10: Pelvic tilt with right knee down

Holding the Legs Up

Many abdominal conditioning exercises call for your legs to be held up in the air, perpendicular to the floor—quite a challenge if you have tight hamstrings or tight back muscles. Let's see if this Feldenkrais-inspired series can help you achieve this position with more comfort.

PILATES EXERCISES

Legs Up and Down, Teaser, 90/90, Inner Thigh Curl, Straight Leg Stretch.

ACTION

Lie on your back and bring both legs straight up in the air. How does that feel? Can you straighten your knees? How long could you stay here?

REPETITIONS

Do 6 to 8 of each of the following instructions. Remember to perform each movement very slowly.

ENHANCING THE ACTION

1. Lie on your back with both feet on the floor and your knees bent. Lift your **right** leg up and hold onto it with both hands. Straighten your **right** knee as much as is comfortable. Bring your nose in the direction of your knee and your knee in the direction of your nose, as though you wanted to touch your nose to your **right** knee. Keep breathing.

2. Now think of bringing your forehead toward your knee and your knee toward your forehead. Exhale as you lift, and inhale as you lower your head.

3. This time have your chin move toward your foot and your foot toward your chin. Are you holding your breath? This time inhale as you lift, and exhale as you lower your head.

4. Change legs, and repeat steps 1 to 3.

5. Lift both feet off the floor and keep your knees bent. Hold your **right** and **left** ankles or lower legs with your hands. Roll just an inch to the **right**, and then to the **left**. Gradually increase the distance you roll.

6. This time straighten your legs in the air as much as possible and hold onto your legs with your hands anywhere that's comfortable. Roll a little to the **right**, and then to the **left.** Increase the range of your side to side movements; but only go so far that you don't find yourself falling or unable to easily return to the center.

7. Stop and rest for a full minute on your back with your legs extended long.

8. Let's see if anything has changed. Bring both legs straight up in the air again. Do you feel it's any easier now?

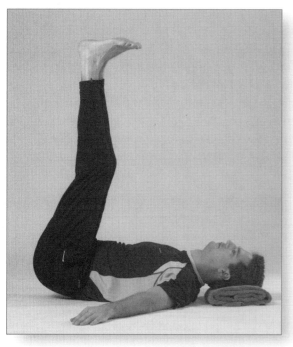

Action: Legs straight up

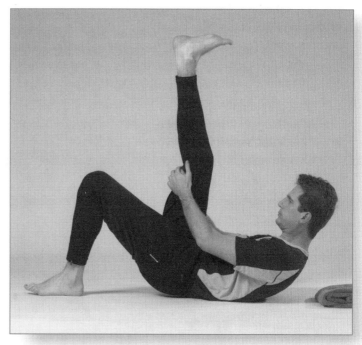

Enhancement No. 2: Right leg up, forehead to knee

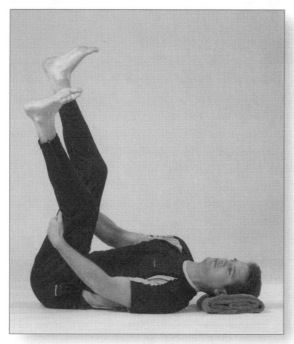

Enhancement No. 6: Legs straight, roll left

Preparing for Back Work I

PURPOSE

We need a strong *and* flexible back to carry us through our daily lives in a fully functional way. Pilates is the perfect approach to achieve this important duality. Use the following sequence to make the back strengthening exercises in this book much easier to perform.

PILATES EXERCISES

Swan, Flight.

ACTION

Lie on your stomach with your hands slightly in front of you and lift your head. How far up can you see without straining? Perhaps you can make a mental mark on a wall in front of you to remind you of where you can see right now.

REPETITIONS

Do 10 repetitions of each step so it is barely perceptible, and then 10 with the intention of increasing the span of each movement, finding a way to make it feel light and easy.

ENHANCING THE ACTION

1. Lie on your stomach with your forehead on your arms, the **right** hand on top of the **left**. Lift your head with your top arm up and down. (Pretend your forehead and **right** hand are "glued" together.) Your **left** arm should remain on the floor.
2. Now lift your head up with your **right** hand and hold it in the air. Begin to slide to the **right** and **left** as if you were dusting the floor with your hand (this is called *translation).* Start *very small* and gradually increase the range of motion, always staying within your comfort zone.
3. Switch hands and turn your head to the other side. Lift your head **up** and **down**, your **left** hand and head glued together.
4. Now lift your head and hand holding them both in the air as you *translate* from **right** to **left**.
5. Stop and rest for a moment. Feel free to lie on your side or on your back.
6. Lie on your stomach and place both hands slightly in front of you. Lift your chin **up** and then **down**.
7. Close your eyes. This time as you lift your chin up look **down** with your eyes. Then lower your chin and look *up* with your eyes.
8. Come back to the initial movement and see if you can lift your head higher than the mark you initially made.

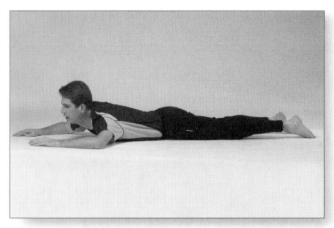

Action: Head lift

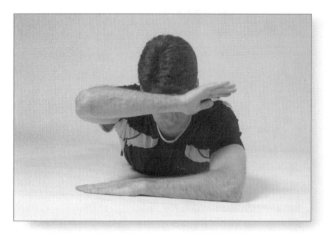

Enhancement No. 1: Right hand on forehead

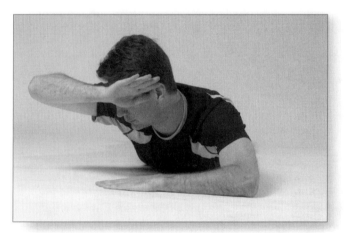

Enhancement No. 2: Right hand on forehead, slide right

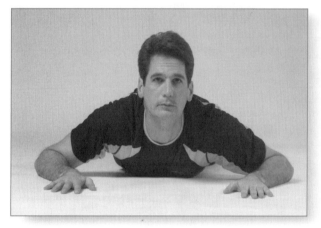

Enhancement No. 6: Chin up

Preparing for Back Work II

PURPOSE

Creating a strong back can be achieved more quickly if we could make other parts of our body, particularly our arms and legs, light and supple.

PILATES EXERCISES

Opposite Arm and Leg Lift, Swimming, Single Leg Lift, Double Leg Lift.

ACTION

Lie on your stomach with your legs long and arms straight out in front of you. Do small "swimming" movements, so that your arms and legs paddle. (See Swimming, page 186).

REPETITIONS

Start with 8 to 10 tiny motions, and gradually increase over the next 8 to 10 repetitions without trying to reach the limit of your ability.

ENHANCING THE ACTION

1. Lie on your *back* with your legs long and spread apart (at least hip distance apart). Have your arms overhead, any place that's comfortable. Raise your **right** leg up, just 1 inch, so that it barely lifts from the floor.
2. Lift your **right** arm up 1 inch from the floor.
3. Now lift your **right** leg and **right** arm up together, just 1 inch from the floor.
4. Do steps 2 and 3 with the left side.
5. Lift your **right** arm and *left* leg up together just a tiny bit from the floor. Can you make it so they lift *precisely* together?
6. Lift your **left** arm and **right** leg up at the exact same moment.
7. Now lie on your *stomach* and do the original movement. Do you feel your body has learned something new?

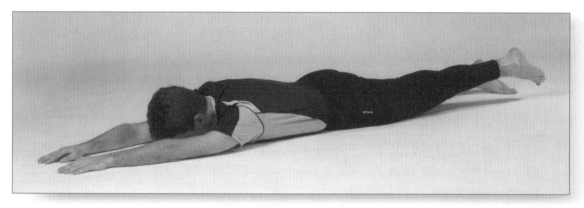

Action: Left leg lift

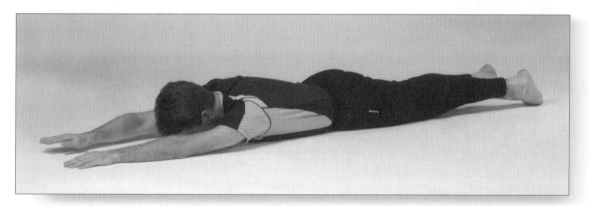

Action: Right arm lift

Breathing

PURPOSE

Breathing empowers the Pilates workout. We are fueled by the oxygen in the air, so the more deeply we breathe, the better we oxygenate and energize our bodies. Here is a quick way to experience a new dimension in your breathing.

PILATES EXERCISES

Every exercise.

ACTION

Lie on your back. Inhale as deeply as you can. How does that feel? What part of you is expanding? Your front, sides, back? Does the air travel upward toward your head or downward toward your feet?

REPETITIONS

Do each instruction very slowly, about 15 times.

ENHANCING THE ACTION

1. As you inhale allow your belly to expand. Exhale and deflate your belly.
2. This time as you inhale pull your belly in. And as you exhale, push your belly out (this is the *opposite* of what you have just been doing.) This may feel impossible right now, but just try and see what happens.
3. Inhale deeply and hold your breath. Still holding your breath, move the air inside up toward your chest, and then down toward your belly. Do it as many times as you can until you have to stop and take a breath. Repeat this several times.
4. Now take a deep breath again. Has anything changed?

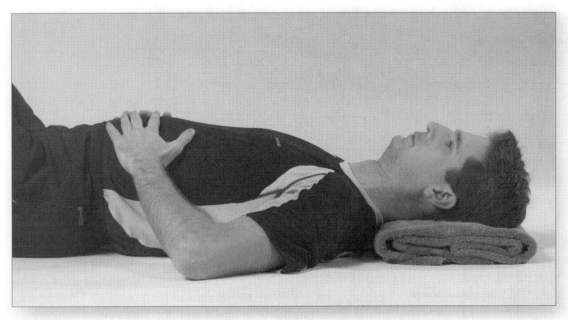

Enhancement No. 1: Inhale with expanded belly

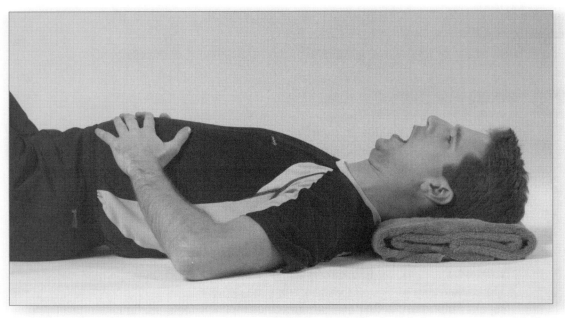

Enhancement No. 2: Exhale with expanded belly

Rolling

PURPOSE

Rolling is a natural and joyful movement, one that all babies and children do effortlessly and gleefully. Bringing some of that playful spirit into adulthood is rejuvenating for the spirit, as well as the body.

PILATES EXERCISES

Rolling Like a Ball.

ACTION

Sit with your knees bent and your chin on your chest. Hold below your knees with your hands. Maintain this tucked position and use momentum to roll down and then back up. How far back can you roll? How smoothly do you roll? (See Rolling Like a Ball for a full explanation of the exercise).

REPETITIONS

Do 4 or 5 of each of the following steps with the least amount of effort possible.

ENHANCING THE ACTION

1. Lie on your back. Hold your knees with your hands. Keep your head on the floor and roll a little to the **right** and then a little to the **left** (just 1 or 2 inches). Imagine there is a stick between your nose and your knees so that they move in total synchrony.
2. Now roll your body to the **right** as you turn your head to the **left**. And roll your body to the **left** as you turn your head to the **right**.
3. This time roll your body to the **right**, turn your head to the **left**, *but move your eyes to the right*. Then do the reverse, roll your knees to the **left**, turn your head to the **right**, *but move your eyes to the left*.
4. Now go back to rolling to the **right** and **left** with your head moving in the same direction as the roll and at exactly the same time.
5. Repeat Rolling like a Ball and see whether it almost feels as though you're flying.

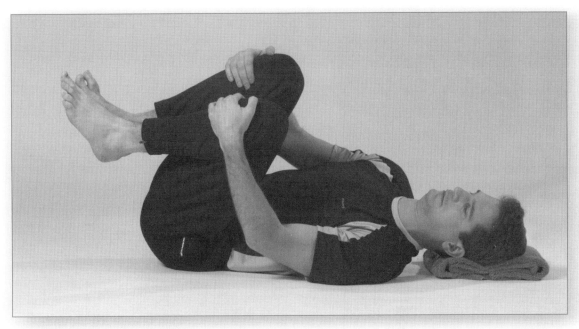

Enhancement No. 1: Roll left

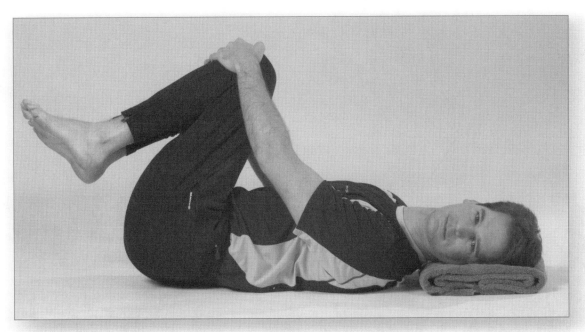

Enhancement No. 2: Knees right, head left

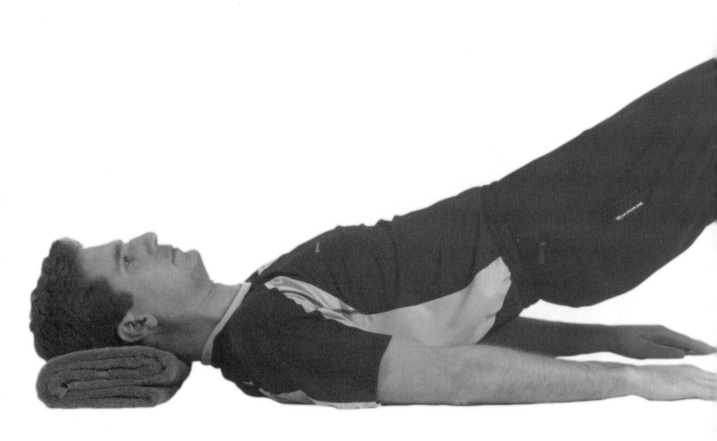

Chapter 7

The Release Movements

The Time In Between

*I*ntegral to the Pilates program are the stretching and lengthening movements interspersed between the power moves. While many may appear familiar to the frequent exerciser, I have given them a Feldenkrais infused "twist" to enhance their value. I call these the "release" movements. Even the advanced Pilates performer will need to take breaks. With any type of sustained effort our muscles produce a harmless by-product called *lactic acid,* which produces a slight burning sensation. This chapter gives you some options to help disperse the lactic acid and allow your body to recover and renew for the next exercise.

Will Resting Diminish Results?

While you will feel it to be a much harder workout if you don't do the release movements, taking these breaks won't detract from the benefits of the exercises. In other words, you can rest and do a release movement between each and every exercise and still reap the same benefits as though you never stopped at all.

Here's why. Pilates is not cardiovascular exercise; it is a program that commingles muscular endurance and flexibility. Continuous, non-stop activity is only required with cardiovascular, or *aerobic*, exercise. Yes, you will most likely sweat more if you never stop and stretch, but the muscle work won't be affected. Your core will still strengthen and your muscles will still lengthen regardless of how often you pause to do a release sequence.

The Benefits of Taking Your Time

You can also use this chapter as a relaxing way to begin or end your day. Just follow the sequences in the order presented. You will immediately reap the benefits of a supple spine, less bodily stiffness, and reduced stress.

For each of the movements that follow feel free to do them as long, or as briefly, as you feel you need. There is no minimum or maximum optimal time. However, you will find that holding each stretch for at least 30 seconds, and performing each movement three or more times will allow your body to move seamlessly into the next progression.

Start small, go slowly, and never feel as though you're straining or pushing. These movements should not hurt at all; you should feel a pleasurable sensation as your muscles relax and lengthen.

Here are the release movements to incorporate into your program:

- Full Body Stretch
- Single Knee to Chest
- Side to Side Rocking
- Circle Knees
- Knees to Floor
- Hip Stretch
- Hip Circles
- Bridge
- Prayer Stretch
- Hip Shake

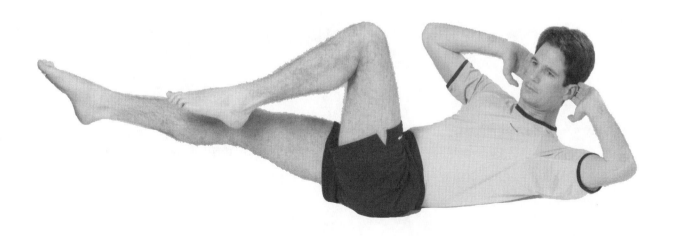

Full Body Stretch

Purpose: To lengthen the spine and stretch the chest and shoulder muscles

1. Lie on your back with your arms overhead and your legs extended long.
2. Reach through your **right** arm and **right** leg simultaneously, as if one person has hold of your **right** wrist and another person has hold of your **right** ankle and they are pulling you apart. Both your arm and leg should remain on the floor.
3. Now as you reach with your **right** arm flex your **right** foot (so your toes come closer to your shin bone).
4. Lift your **left** hip up toward your head so that your side bends a little to the **left**; think of "hiking up" your **left** hip. Be sure your back and pelvis stay on the floor.
5. Repeat the hiking motion and allow your head to move where it naturally wants to go.
6. Finally, reach with your **right** arm and leg and at the same time turn your head to look at your **right** hand.
7. Perform steps 2 to 6 with your **left** arm and **left** leg.

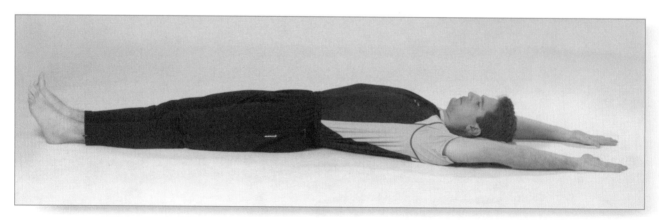

Step No. 1: Arms overhead, legs extended

Single Knee to Chest

Purpose: To stretch the lower back

1. Lie on your back with your legs extended long. Bring your **right** knee into your chest and pull it in with your arms.
2. Place your **left** hand on your breastbone and gently slide it down in the direction of your feet (not in the direction of the floor).
3. Place your **left** hand on your lower ribs and gently guide them in the direction of your stomach.
4. Repeat the above with your **left** knee held into your chest.

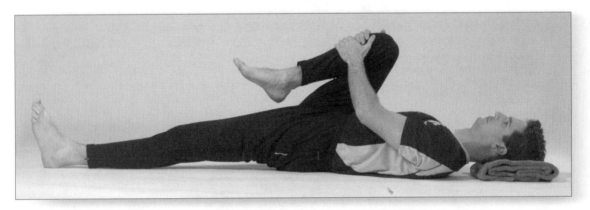

Step No. 1: Right knee to chest

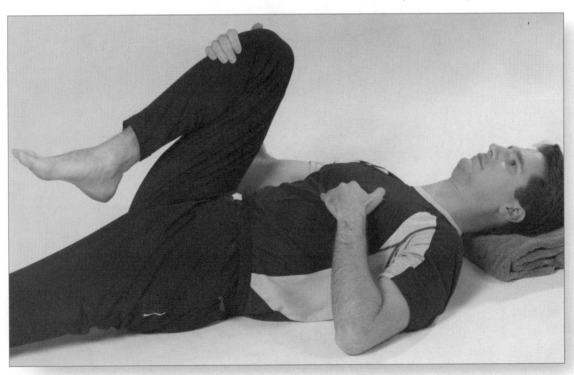

Step No. 2: Breastbone slide down

Side to Side Rocking

Purpose: To stretch the lower back

1. Lie on your back and lift both knees toward your chest. Pull your knees farther in with your arms.
2. Lengthen the back of your neck so your chin comes a little closer to your chest.
3. Soften your chest and relax your rib cage so it moves downward toward your stomach.
4. Rock side to side, still holding onto your legs, and allow your head to move freely in the same direction as your legs.
5. Now move your knees to the **right** as your turn your head to the **left**. Then reverse that so your knees move to the **left** as you turn your head to the **right**.
6. Come back to rocking side to side again and allow your head to move **right** and **left** in the same direction as your legs.

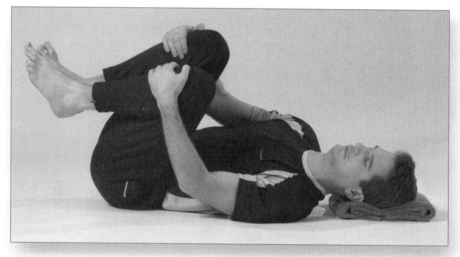

Step No. 4: Rock side to side

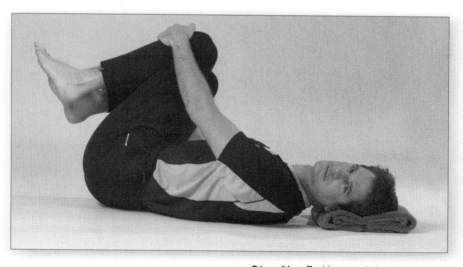

Step No. 5: Knees right, head left

Circle Knees

Purpose: To reduce neck and back tension

1. Lie on your back with both knees pulled into your chest, holding below your knees lightly with your hands.
2. Make a big circle with your knees and allow your head to freely join in the movement.
3. Change the direction of the knee circles and allow your head to join in the movement.

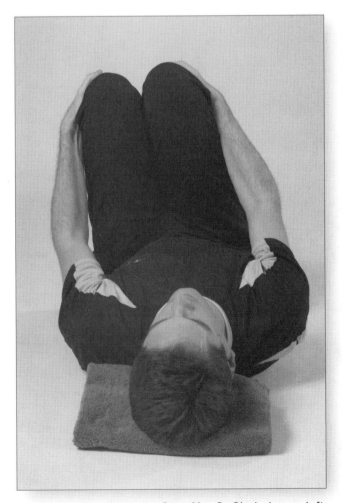

Step No. 2: Circle knees left

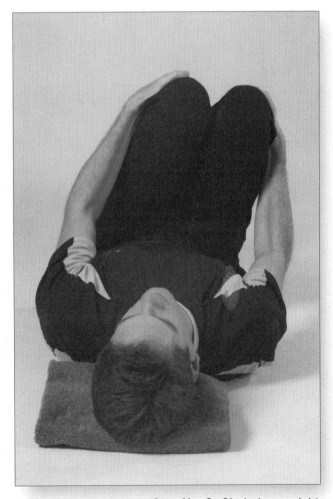

Step No. 3: Circle knees right

Knees to Floor

Purpose: To stretch the back, hip, and chest

1. Lie on your back with both knees pulled into your chest and your arms out to your side.
2. Slowly let both knees fall to the **left**, all the way to the floor if possible. Keep your **right** arm on the floor if you can do so without straining. Relax your feet, your knees, and your inner thighs.
3. Slide your **right** arm up along the floor toward your head, and then back down a few times. Feel the additional stretch in your chest as your arm comes towards your head.
4. This time slide your **right** arm up along the floor toward your head and keep it at the highest comfortable position. Lift your **right** hip a little so your pelvis rolls to the **left** and increases the stretch along your **right** chest area.
5. Change sides. Let both knees fall to the **right** and repeat steps 3 and 4 using your **left** arm.

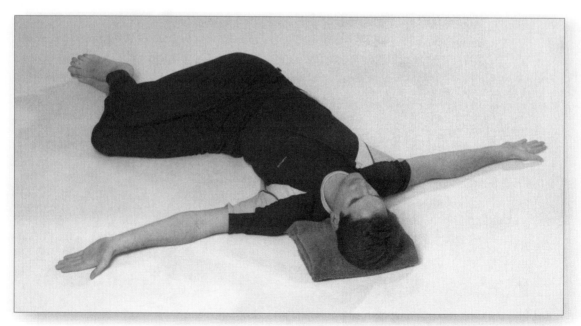

Step No. 2: Arms out, knees left

Hip Stretch

Purpose: To stretch the buttocks and lower back

1. Lie on your back, lift your knees toward your chest and cross your **right** leg over the **left**, with your **right** knee turned out. Move your legs slightly to the **left**. Use your arms to pull your legs in closer to your body and hold this stretch before proceeding.
2. Turn your head to the **right** and hold it there.
3. Then turn your head to the **left** and hold it here.
4. Change legs, and repeat all of the above.

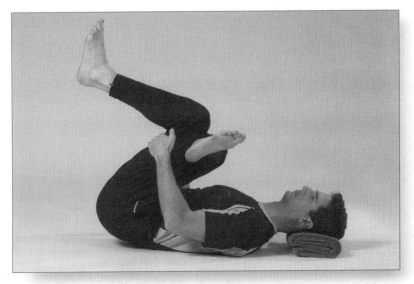

Step No. 1: Right knee turned out

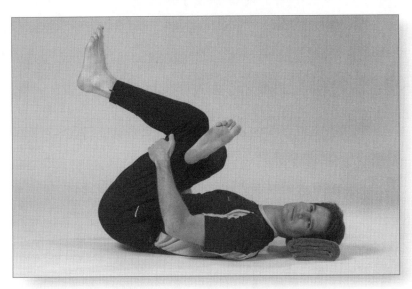

Step No. 3: Head turn left

Hip Circles

Purpose: To stretch the buttocks and reduce lower back tension

1. Lie on your back with your knees pulled into your chest. Cross your **right** leg over the left, and turn your **right** knee out to the side.
2. Circle both knees to the **right** several times, allowing your head to participate in the circle.
3. Circle to the **left**.
4. Change legs and repeat steps 2 and 3.

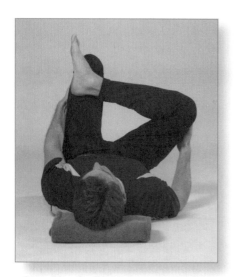

Step No. 1: Right knee turned out

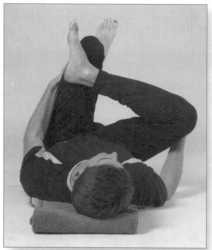

Step No. 2: Knees circle right, head moves

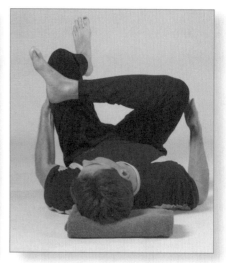

Step No. 3: Knees circle left, head moves

Bridge

Purpose: To stretch the abdominals and hip flexors

1. Lie on your back with both feet flat on the floor.
2. Slowly lift your hips up so that your spine comes off the floor, peeling up one vertebra at a time. Then slowly lower so that, one after the other, each vertebra touches the floor.
3. Lift your hips up and down as you turn your head to the **right** and **left**.
4. Keep your head turning independently from the movement in your lower body so that your head turns at one speed and your lower body lifts and lowers at another.

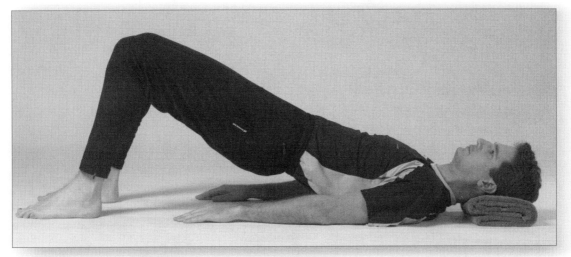

Step No. 2: Hip lift

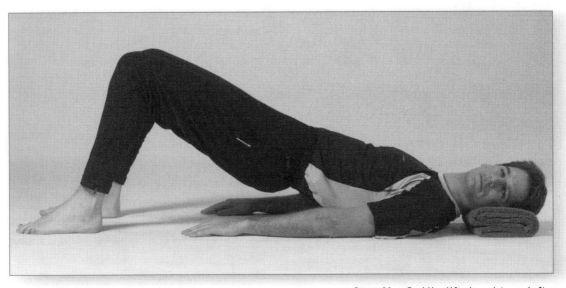

Step No. 3: Hip lift, head turn left

Prayer Stretch

Purpose: To stretch the backs of the arms and the upper, middle, and lower back

1. Rest on your knees and bend over so your arms are outstretched in front of you.
2. Walk your hands out in front of you as far as you can.
3. Walk your hands to the **left** as you sink into your **right** hip.
4. Then, walk your hands to the **right** as you sink into your **left** hip.

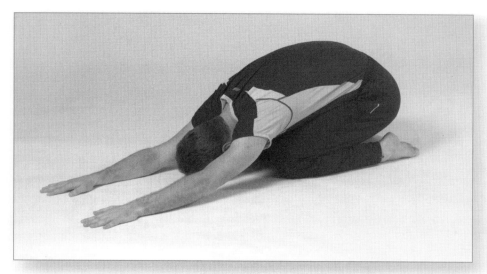

Step No. 1: Arms outstretched overhead

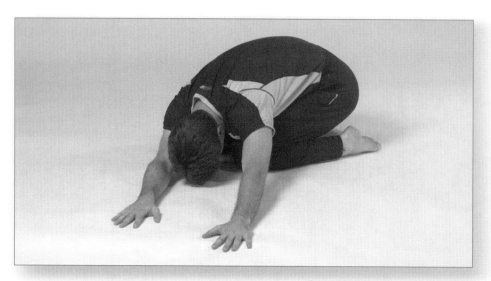

Step No. 3: Hands walk left

Hip Shake

Purpose: To reduce tension in the lower back

1. Lie on your stomach with your head on your arms in a comfortable position.
2. Shake your hips very slightly to the **right** and **left** a few times.
3. Increase the range of movement so that your hips (first the **right** and then the **left**) lift slightly off the floor.

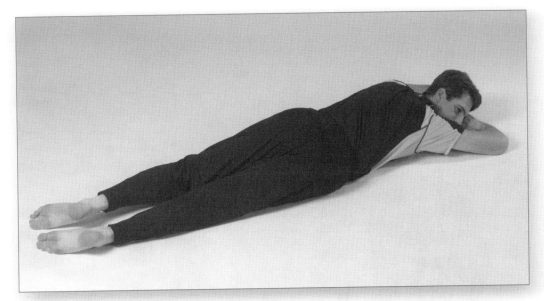

Step No. 1: Hip shake right

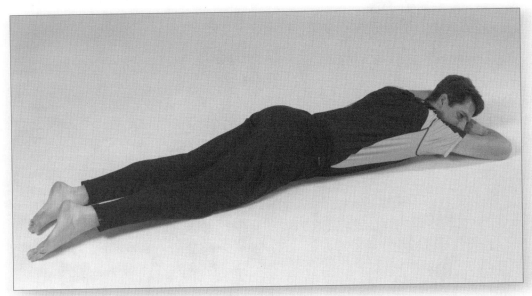

Step No. 2: Raised hip shake left

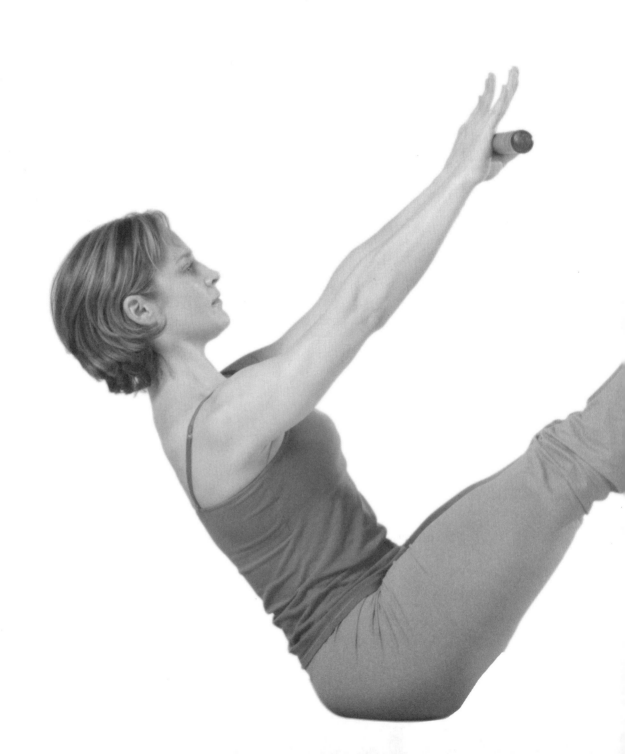

Chapter 8

The Mat Exercises

Building Up From the Foundation

*T*o truly practice the Pilates method, you must immediately incorporate *all* of the basic principles. Have you reviewed Chapter 4: *Learning the Basics* and Chapter 5: *Form and Alignment?* If not, please do so for they will help you gain the understanding and control essential to the Pilates discipline. And take a look at Chapter 6: *The Secrets to Good Pilates Technique,* to become more aware of your body's potential to overcome restrictions that may deter from your performance.

If you're a beginner you will find Chapter 4: *Learning The Basics* an excellent introductory program and, when combined with Chapter 6, you will enjoy a new appreciation of your body's ability to move. Even intermediate or advanced students will make discoveries that enhance their experience. Take the time to become acquainted or reacquainted with the framework that makes Pilates so unique.

Choosing the Right Mat Exercises for You

As you will see, each Mat exercise has a level assigned to it: Beginner, Intermediate, or Advanced. It's always wise to initiate a new exercise program with Beginner level exercises before moving up to more difficult ones.

There will be *Prerequisite* instruction referring you to a Basic move or previous Mat exercise. For your safety and comfort, be sure you can accomplish these before attempting the exercise on the page.

You'll profit by doing any of the *Enhancements* listed. These have their inspiration from the Feldenkrais philosophy and are included to make your Pilates experience more esthetic, productive, and pleasurable.

Pay close attention to the *Starting Position*. This will generally also be the position to which you return after each repetition. Read the description of the *Action* phase and go over the *Body Check* elements two or three times before attempting to perform any of the exercises.

Always feel free to choose the *Power It Down* option if you are straining in any way. Pilates seeks inner strength that gets projected outward so movements are always fluid and graceful while appearing effortless.

As you internalize the Pilates basics and feel more conditioned you may want to try the *Power It Up* suggestions. These will either increase the range of motion of the exercise or incorporate resistance (e.g., ankle or wrist weights) to your core conditioning. In addition to increasing the intensity of the exercise, the additional equipment further shapes and defines your arm and leg muscles. A beginner exercise can become more advanced when *Power It Up* ideas are used.

Breathing is Key

Inhale through your nose and exhale through your mouth. With each inhalation you lengthen and expand all three dimensions of your rib cage, front, side, and back. You may be asked to reach through your fingers, your legs, your heels, or out of your waist. Feel that you are getting taller, being stretched out, or increasing the space between each vertebra.

With each exhalation pay attention to your core to support your entire body. Every time you expel air bring your navel to your spine and perform a Kegel. Use your power of visualization to "see" your lungs fully expand and then thoroughly deflate as all the air is squeezed out.

Use your breath to put power into your execution; to access your internal musculature; to keep your focus and concentration and to help you do just one more repetition. Use your breath and you will find yourself continually progressing and improving. It is one of the indispensable tools to unearth and bring forth your body's untapped power.

Interspersing "Strength" with "Length"

As described in Chapter 7: *The Release Movements* reduce tension that normally develops during intense exercise and also improve flexibility. Initially I recommend you do a release movement after each exercise. As you advance you can choose whether to take this time between exercises. Because they lengthen and stretch the body, the release movements add value to your workout.

Before You Begin

Use a well-cushioned mat. Lying on your side or putting weight on your knees can be uncomfortable for some people without this added padding.

Take a moment to perceive your head alignment when you are on your back (see page 52) in case you need to put something under your head to elevate it a little bit from the floor.

Be sure you warm up before starting your Pilates workout so that you can fully benefit from the program. In order for your muscles to fully benefit from the exercises they need to be warm and limber; your blood needs to be pumping through them.

Quality, Not Quantity

Your primary goal is always to condition the core. Therefore, as long as you feel that you are working with inner intensity it is not necessary to achieve the range of motion the picture may portray. The issue is never how much, but *how well.* A small range of motion or fewer repetitions is far superior when done with concentration, proper breathing, and strict adherence to the instructions. Attend to *all* the elements delineated in the *Body Check* category to make your Pilates experience pay off.

The progression of exercises in this chapter allows you to complete a series on your back, then seated, then on your hands and knees, and finally on your stomach. Also built into the sequence design is consideration of the exercise intensity. After a few strenuous moves, the focus will shift to another muscle group. This gives the muscles you were just working a chance to recuperate.

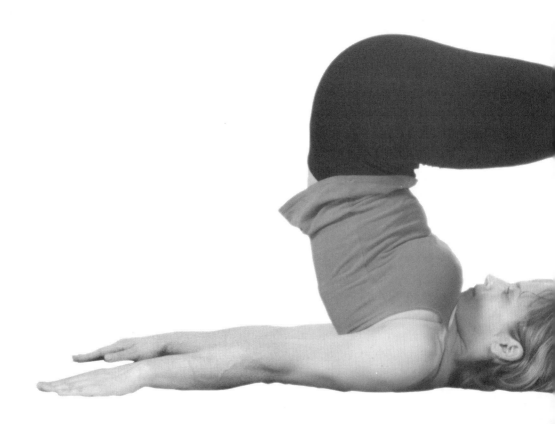

Here is the Pilates Mat repetoire:

- Breathing to 100
- Roll Up
- Single Knee Stretch
- Double Leg Extension
- Straight Leg Stretch
- 90/90
- Pilates First
- Inner Thigh Curl
- Buttocks Squeeze
- Legs Lower and Lift
- Teaser I
- Teaser II
- Leg Circles
- Crisscross
- Scissors
- Rollover
- Spine Stretch
- Seated Twist
- Rolling Like A Ball
- Roll Down

- Reverse Hold
- Leg Pull Front
- Side Leg Series
- Side Stretch
- Mermaid
- Push-Up Hold
- Leg Pull Back
- Push-Ups
- 4 Points
- 4 Points Leg Series
- Swan
- Flight
- Opposite Arm and Leg Lift
- Swimming
- Double Leg Lift
- Quad Stretch
- Rocking
- Cat Stretch

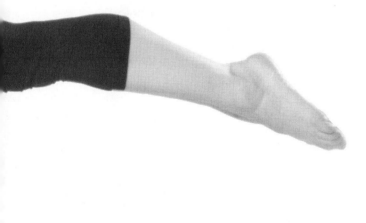

Breathing to 100

Level	Beginner
Purpose	Circulate oxygen and blood to the muscles and isometrically strengthen the abdominals
Prerequisites	Deep Abdominal Contraction, page 41; Engaging the Lats, page 44
Enhancements	Holding the Head Up, page 68; Shoulders Up and Down, page 78

THE EXERCISES

Starting Position	Lie on your back with your feet on the floor. Your arms should be by your sides with palms down.
Action	Lift your head and allow your arms to lift a few inches off the floor. Reach out through your hands as if to touch a wall in front of you. Hold this position as you inhale for 5 counts, and exhale for 5 counts, until you reach a total of 100 counts.
Repetitions	100 counts, which will be 10 inhales and 10 exhales

BODY CHECK

Head	Do not look up at the ceiling. Your chin should be tilting slightly down, not up.
Shoulders	Gently pull your shoulders down by Engaging The Lats.
Arms/Hands	Keep reaching through your hands as if to touch a wall in front of you.
Pelvis	Stabilize your pelvis with a Deep Abdominal Contraction; do not tuck your pelvis under or allow your hips to move at all.
Legs	Place your feet slightly forward of your knees.
Feet	Your feet should be relaxed.

You Are Doing It Correctly if you feel the work in your abdominals, you are breathing deeply, *and* you continue to keep your head and neck relaxed.

VARIATIONS

Power It Up	Bring your legs straight up in the air so they are perpendicular to the floor. Move your hands in a small up and down pressing movement, about 3 inches in each direction. Inhale as you "pump" up and down 5 times, and then exhale for 5 pumps. The challenge is to stabilize your spine so that it is anchored into the floor and does not move at all. These are the traditional Pilates "Hundreds."

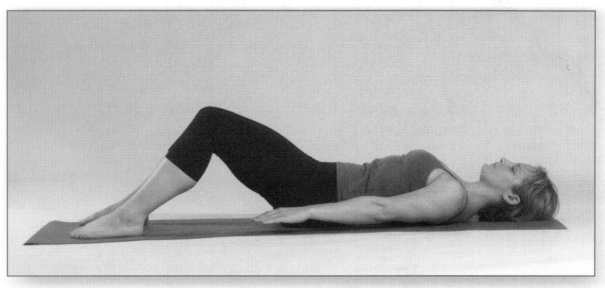

Starting Position: Head down, arms by sides

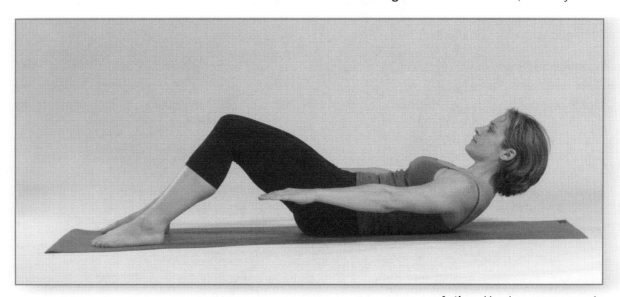

Action: Head up, arms reach

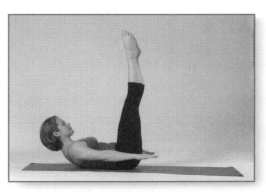

Power It Up: Legs straight up

Roll Up

Level	Beginner
Purpose	Abdominal strengthening
Prerequisite	Breathing to 100, page 120
Enhancement	Arms Lying Straight Overhead, page 80

THE EXERCISES

Starting Position
Lie on your back with your legs extended on the floor, feet flexed, and arms overhead.

Action
Exhale as you bring your arms over to your mid-chest area. Now lift your head off the floor and reach your arms forward, but keep your lower back in contact with the floor. Inhale and return to starting position.

Repetitions
Perform 8 times.

BODY CHECK

Head
Keep your head and neck free from tension. Allow your chin to come nearer to your chest.

Shoulders
Your shoulders should remain down.

Arms/Hands
Reach through your fingers as though to touch an imaginary wall in front of you.

Pelvis
The challenge is to stabilize your pelvis. You will feel a tendency for your lower back to press down into the floor, which means your pelvis has tilted. Counteract this by engaging your abdominals fully and using your breath to bring your navel to your spine. If you come up too high you will use your hip flexor muscles and not your abdominal muscles.

Legs
Tighten your buttocks and upper part of your outer thighs to turn your legs out from your hips. Strive to keep your legs from moving at all.

Feet
Gently flex your feet, reaching through your heels.

You Are Doing It Correctly if you bring your arms up first and then lift your head up *and* if you curl up smoothly with no unevenness or jerky motions.

VARIATIONS

Power It Down
Keep your knees bent and your feet on the floor.

Power It Up
Keep your arms overhead as you curl up so your head and arms lift simultaneously. For maximum challenge, hold a body bar or strap on wrist weights.

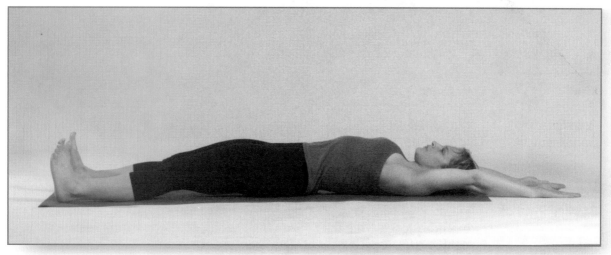

Starting Position: Arms overhead, head down

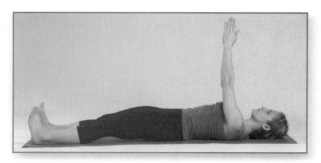

Action: Arms raised, head down

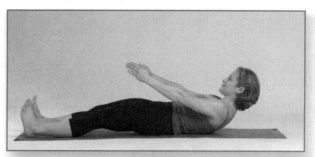

Action: Arms raised, head up

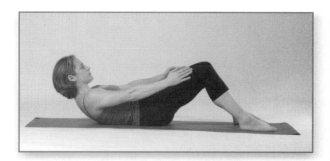

Power It Down: Knees bent

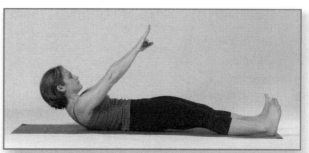

Power It Up: Using Body Bar

Single Knee Stretch

Level	Beginner
Purpose	Isometric abdominal toning
Prerequisite	Roll Up, page 122
Enhancement	Single Knee to Chest, page 105

THE EXERCISES

Starting Position Lie on your back with your **right** knee bent into your chest and your **left** leg extended long on the floor. Place both hands, touching lightly, just below your **right** knee. Lift your head off the floor.

Action Keep your head lifted as you switch legs so your **left** knee comes into your chest and your **right** leg extends straight about 2 inches off the floor. (Your straightened leg should stay off the floor each time). Breathe in for two leg stretches (one **right** and one **left**) and then out for two.

Repetitions Perform 8 sets (right and left counts as 1 set).

BODY CHECK

Head	Think of bringing your nose toward your knee.
Shoulders	Pull your shoulder blades down.
Arms/Hands	Keep your hands and arms light and relaxed.
Pelvis	Fully anchor your body; your spine and pelvis should not move at all. Strongly pull your navel in toward your spine.
Legs	Keep lengthening the leg that is extending (straightening).
Feet	Gently point your foot.

You Are Doing It Correctly if you feel your extended leg is being pulled out of its hip socket *and* you feel the work of the exercise occurring deep within your belly.

VARIATIONS

Power It Down	Don't extend your legs fully; keep your knees slightly bent.
Power It Up	Use ankle weights.

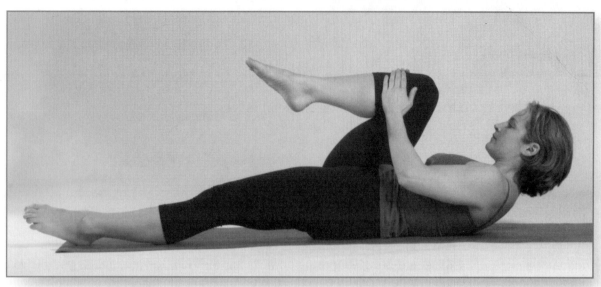

Starting Position: Right knee to chest, head up. *Correct position is leg 2 inches off the floor.*

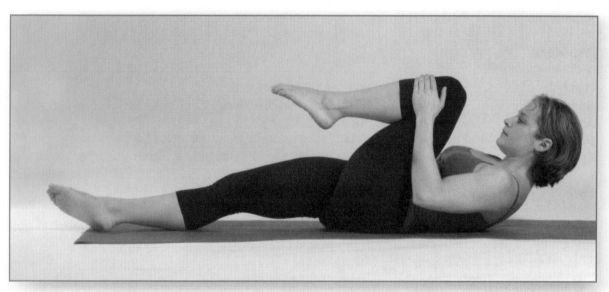

Action: Left knee to chest, right leg lift. *Correct position is leg 2 inches off the floor.*

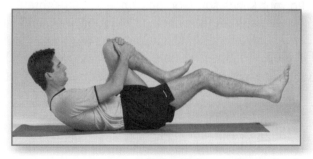

Power It Down: Knees bent

Double Leg Extension

Level	Intermediate
Purpose	Strengthen and tone the abdominals
Prerequisite	Single Knee Stretch, page 124
Enhancement	Holding the Head Up, page 68

THE EXERCISES

Starting Position   Lie on your back with your knees bent and feet off the floor. Bring both arms out to the sides, palms up.

Action   Exhale and bring your arms down along the floor to your legs as you lift your head off the floor. Try to come up to where you are balanced on your tailbone. Inhale and return to starting position.

Repetitions   Perform 8 times.

BODY CHECK

Head	Keep your head and neck light and relaxed.
Shoulders	Use your lats to keep your shoulders down.
Arms/Hands	Reach through your arms and hands to enable you to lift higher.
Pelvis	Feel the work emanating from your abdominal muscles.
Legs	Begin with your knees and lower legs together. Then straighten your legs, lengthening them out of the hip sockets.
Feet	Gently point your feet.

You Are Doing It Correctly if you do not use momentum *and* initiate the work from deep within your abdominal wall.

VARIATIONS

Power It Down   Keep your knees soft (you don't need to straighten them all the way). Curl up so you are still on your back, and not on your tailbone.

Power It Up   Use ankle weights and hold a body bar over your chest. Press the bar away from your chest so your elbows straighten ("bench press") as you extend your legs and come up to balance on your pelvis.

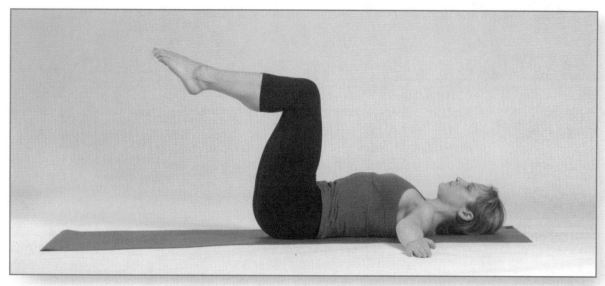

Starting Position: Knees bent, legs raised

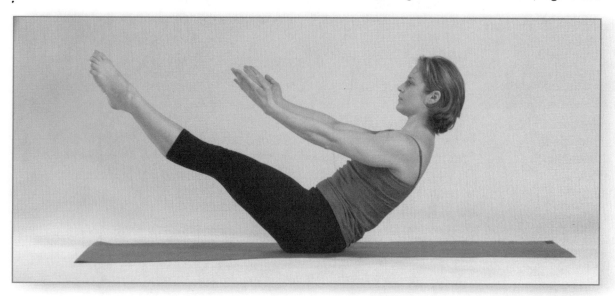

Action: Balance on pelvis, legs straight

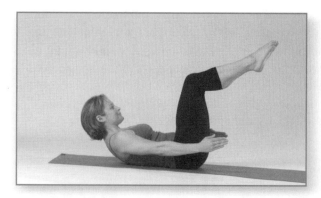

Power It Down: Balance on back, knees bent

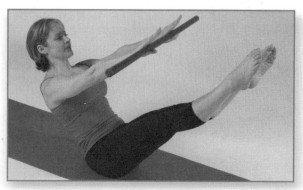

Power It Up: Balance on pelvis with Body Bar

Straight Leg Stretch

Level	Intermediate
Purpose	Isometric abdominal strengthening, hamstring flexibility
Prerequisites	Single Knee Stretch, page 124
	See Power It Down at bottom of this page for hamstring stretch
Enhancement	Hamstring Flexibility, page 84

THE EXERCISES

Starting Position	Hold onto your **right** leg, keeping it as straight as you can, and extend your **left** leg.
Action	Switch legs so you pull your **left** leg toward your chest and extend your **right** leg long, keeping it 2 inches off the floor. Keep the extended leg off the floor each time you switch legs. Inhale for one set and exhale for the next.
Repetitions	Perform 8 sets (right and left count as 1 set).

BODY CHECK

Head	Keep your head and neck relaxed.
Shoulders	Use your lats to keep your shoulders down.
Arms/Hands	Your hands and arms should stay soft as you gently pull your leg in.
Pelvis	Fully anchor your body; your spine and pelvis should not move at all.
Legs	Squeeze the side of your buttocks to turn your legs out, and feel them moving out of the hip joints and lengthening.
Feet	Gently point your feet.

You Are Doing It Correctly if you are holding your head and torso still *and* feel intense work in your abdominals.

VARIATIONS

Power It Down	If you have very tight hamstrings, then start with this stretch. Place a towel under your **right** foot so you can hold onto either end. Keep your **left** leg extended long on the floor and pull with the towel to bring your **right** leg up as high as you can. The back of your neck should remain lengthened and relaxed on the floor. Inhale deeply and exhale fully 10 times, with each breath moving your leg half and inch closer to you. (You can also put your leg inside a Magic Ring). After performing this stretch, try the exercise again.
Power It Up	Strap on ankle weights.

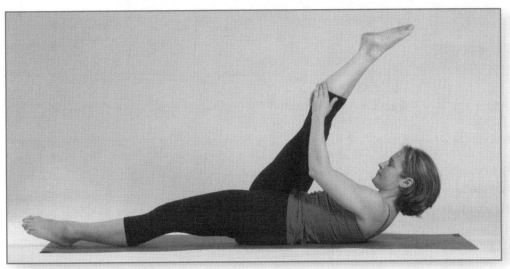

Starting Position: Right leg to chest. *Correct position for left leg is 2 inches off the floor.*

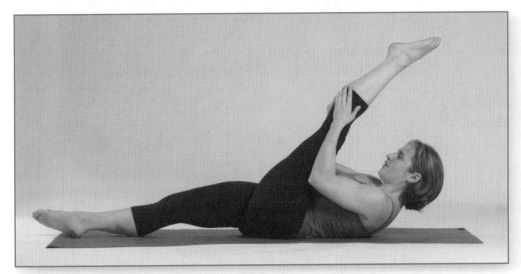

Action: Left leg to chest. *Correct position for right leg is 2 inches off the floor.*

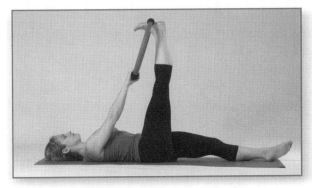

Power It Down: Right leg pull with Magic Ring

90/90

AT A GLANCE

Level	Intermediate
Purpose	Strengthen and tone the abdominals
Prerequisite	Straight Leg Stretch, page 128
Enhancements	Holding the Legs Up, page 90; Arms Lying Straight Overhead, page 80

THE EXERCISES

Starting Position
Lie on your back with your legs up in the air, knees as straight as possible, feet pointed, and arms overhead. Turn your legs out by squeezing the sides of your buttocks muscles and the backs of your upper legs.

Action
Exhale as you do a Deep Abdominal Contraction and bring your arms up to your mid-chest area. Now, lift your head off the floor and curl up. Bring your arms parallel to the floor. Inhale and return to the starting position.

Repetitions
Perform 8 times.

BODY CHECK

Head
Keep your head and neck free of tension. Move your arms first; only when they are over your chest should you lift your head.

Shoulders
As you move your arms over your chest, engage your lats so that your shoulder blades move downward.

Arms/Hands
When your arms are overhead and resting on the floor, focus on lengthening out of your waist by reaching through your fingers.

Pelvis
Bring your navel to your spine and perform a Kegel to deeply contract your abdominals.

Legs
Remember that your legs should not turn out from your feet. Your feet should turn out *as a result of* the external rotation at your hip.

Feet
Gently point your feet out.

You Are Doing It Correctly if you feel tension *only* in your abdominals *and* the rest of your body feels relaxed.

VARIATIONS

Power It Down
When your legs are in the air, keep your knees bent.

Power It Up
Place a Magic Ring between your legs.

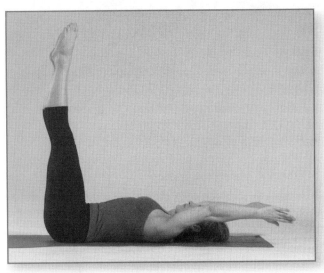

Starting Position: Legs straight up

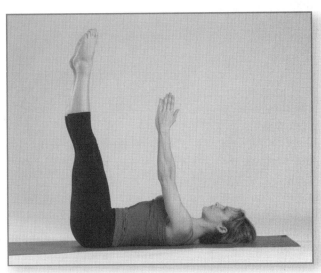

Action: Arms raised

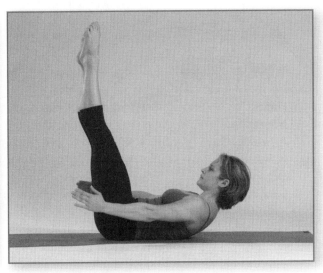

Action: Arms parallel to floor, head raised

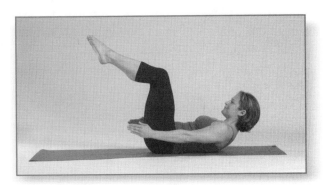

Power It Down: Knees bent

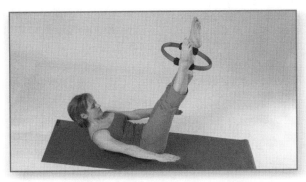

Power It Up: Magic Ring between legs

Pilates First

Level	Intermediate
Purpose	Tone the inner thighs; strengthen the abdominals
Prerequisite	Turning Out From the Hip, page 54
Enhancement	Inner Thigh Flexibility, page 86

THE EXERCISES

Starting Position Lie on your back and bring the soles of your feet together with your knees wide open. Your arms should be out to the sides, palms up.

Action Exhale as you (1) bring your arms down by your sides (2) straighten your legs (3) turn your legs out by squeezing the sides of your buttocks (4) flex your feet and (5) lift your head off the floor. Inhale and return to the starting position.

Repetitions Perform 10 times.

BODY CHECK

Head	Keep your head and neck free of tension.
Shoulders	Gently press your shoulder blades down.
Arms/Hands	Reach with your hands, palms up, as though to touch a wall in front of you.
Pelvis	Pull your navel to your spine and perform a Kegel with each exhalation.
Legs	Squeeze the sides of your buttocks to turn your legs out from your hips.
Feet	Gently flex your feet and press out through your heels.

You Are Doing It Correctly if you maintain focus on your abdominals so that the work is concentrated in your mid-section.

VARIATIONS

Power It Down Move your legs *without* lifting your head off the floor.

Power It Up Add ankle weights and do a "bench press" with a body bar. Start with the bar over your chest and press it away from your chest as you lift your head off the floor.

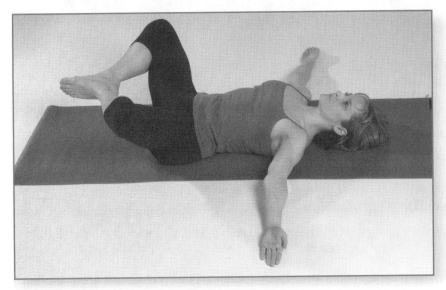

Starting Position: Soles together, knees spread

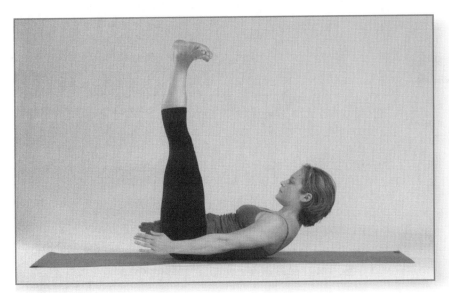

Action: Legs straight, head up

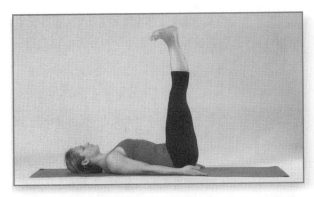

Power It Down: Legs straight, head down

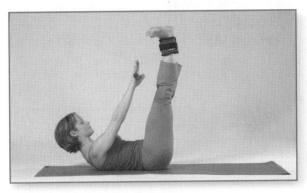

Power It Up: Bench press using ankle weights

Inner Thigh Curl

Level	Intermediate
Purpose	Tone the inner thighs, strengthen the abdominals
Prerequisites	Pointing and Flexing the Foot, page 57; Turning Out From the Hip, page 54
Enhancement	Inner Thigh Flexibility, page 86

THE EXERCISES

Starting Position	Lie on your back and open your legs as wide as you comfortably can. Turn your legs out and flex your feet.
Action	Exhale as you bring your legs together (keeping them turned out), point your feet, and lift your head off the floor. Inhale and return to the starting position.
Repetitions	Perform 10 times.

BODY CHECK

Head	Keep your head and neck free of tension.
Shoulders	Gently press your shoulder blades down.
Arms/Hands	Reach with your hands, palms up, as if to touch a wall in front of you.
Pelvis	With each exhale perform a Deep Abdominal Contraction.
Legs	Do not "bounce" when you open your legs. Stay in control and don't try to force a stretch. Turn your legs out from your hips.
Feet	Flex by pressing through your heels, and point by stretching the arch on the top of your feet.

You Are Doing It Correctly if you deeply contract your abdominals *and* you open and close your legs slowly without bouncing at the bottom.

VARIATIONS

Power It Down	Move your legs *without* lifting your head off the floor.
Power It Up	Add ankle weights and come up to balance on your tailbone.

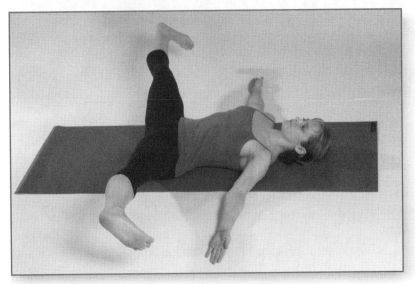

Starting Position: Legs spread

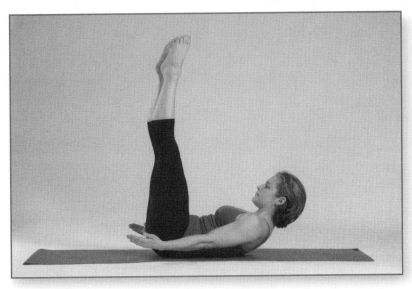

Action: Legs together, head up

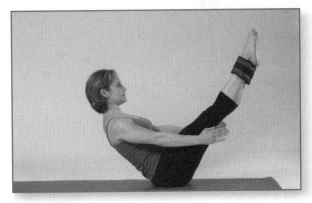

Power It Up: Balance on pelvis with ankle weights

Buttocks Squeeze

Level	Beginner
Purpose	Tone the buttocks and inner thigh muscles; strengthen the abdominals and pelvic floor
Prerequisite	Pelvic Tilt, page 70
Enhancement	Bridge, page 111

THE EXERCISES

Starting Position	Lie on your back and place a Magic Ring* between your knees. Lift your hips off the floor.
Action	Exhale and lift your hips up 2 or 3 inches more. At the same time do a Deep Abdominal Contraction, squeeze your buttocks, and squeeze the Magic Ring. Inhale and lower your hips about 3 inches.
Repetitions	Squeeze and release 20 times.

BODY CHECK

Head	Your neck should be lengthened with your chin down.
Shoulders	Keep them down and relaxed.
Arms/Hands	Your palms should stay on the floor, hands reaching toward your heels.
Pelvis	Use your breathing to make all the pelvic and buttocks contractions deeper. Be sure to only lower your hips about 3 inches.
Legs	Your knees should be at least 12 inches apart.
Feet	Your feet should be about 12 inches apart. Make sure your feet support your body weight, not the back of your neck.

You Are Doing It Correctly if you feel your abdominals working *and* a stretch along your inner thighs.

* Or you can use a small stability ball, medicine ball, or large towel.

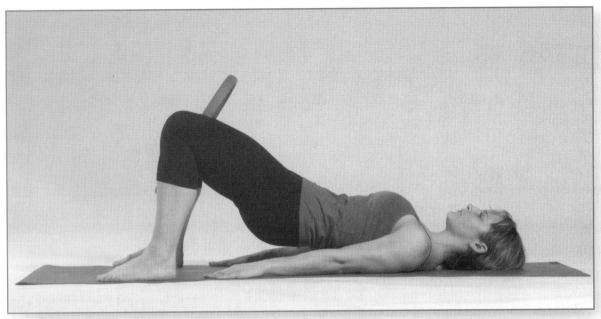

Starting Position: Hips raised

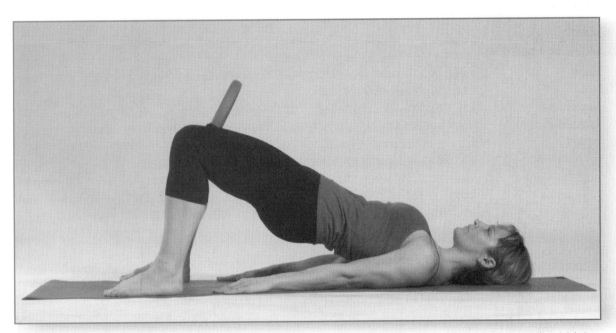

Action: Hips raised higher

Legs Lower and Lift

AT A GLANCE

Level	Advanced
Purpose	Strengthen the lower fibers of the abdominals
Prerequisites	90/90, page 130; Straight Leg Stretch, page 128
Enhancements	Holding the Head Up, page 68; Holding the Legs Up, page 90

THE EXERCISES

Starting Position Lie on your back with your legs in the air directly over your hips. Turn your legs out from your hips with your feet pointed. Place your hands behind your head. Raise your head and hold it there throughout the exercise.

Action Inhale and lower your legs down about 6 inches. Exhale and return to the starting position. Do not allow your legs to come closer to your chest on the return. (If you feel pain in your back, stop immediately).

Repetitions Perform 5 times.

BODY CHECK

Head Keep your head raised throughout the exercise. If you need to lower your head, use the *Power It Down* option.

Shoulders Engage your lats to keep your shoulders down.

Arms/Hands Your fingers should lightly touch the back of your head.

Pelvis Do not allow your lower back to arch or come away from the floor. Use your abdominals to maintain pelvic stabilization.

Legs Turn your legs out from your hips. Your legs should return to the starting position directly over your hips, and not over your chest. If you feel your abdominals relax, you have brought your legs too far toward your chest on the return.

Feet Gently point your feet.

You Are Doing It Correctly if your entire body remains relaxed with tension only occurring in your abdominals

VARIATIONS

Power It Down Bend your knees in the air. Do one repetition, place both feet on the floor and let your head come to rest on the floor for a moment. Return to the starting position, knees bent, and repeat.

Power It Up Increase the distance you lower your legs *as long as* you can maintain pelvic and spinal stabilization. Your lower back should not arch off the floor at all. You can also place a Magic Ring between your lower legs.

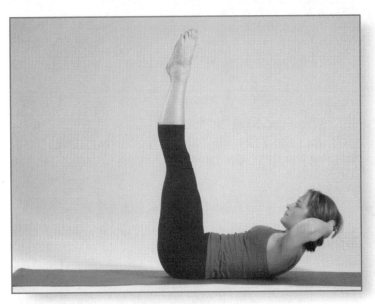

Starting Position: Legs straight, head up

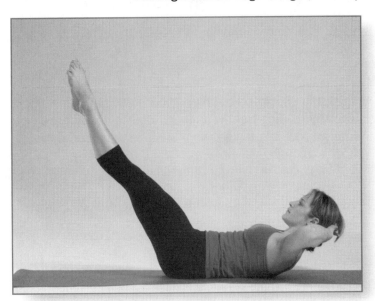

Action: Legs lowered, head up

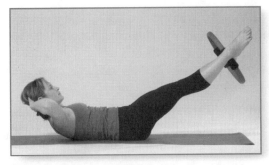

Power It Up: Legs lowered further, head up

Teaser I

Level	Intermediate
Purpose	Strengthen and tone the abdominals
Prerequisite	Roll Up, page 122
Enhancement	Holding the Head Up, page 68

THE EXERCISES

Starting Position
Lie on your back with your arms overhead and both feet flat on the floor. Keep both knees aligned or "glued" together as you straighten just your **left** leg.

Action
Inhale and lengthen through your arms. Exhale and bring your arms over your mid-chest and then lift your head off the floor. Come up to balance on your tailbone with your arms parallel to your extended **left** leg.

Repetitions
Perform 5 times with your left leg up, then switch legs.

BODY CHECK

Head
Your chin should be down and your head and neck should be free of tension. Think of leading from your chest, not from your head.

Shoulders
Engage your lats to keep your shoulders pressed down.

Arms/Hands
Reach through your fingers to lengthen out of your waist when your arms are overhead, and reach again through your fingers when your head is off the floor in the curled up position.

Pelvis
Your goal is to access the deepest layers of your abdominals. Use the Deep Abdominal Contraction and your breathing.

Legs
Your extended leg should be in the Pilates stance, which is turned out at the hip.

Feet
Gently point your foot.

You Are Doing It Correctly if you are performing slow and controlled movements without flinging your body upwards.

VARIATIONS

Power It Down
Curl up as much as you can. You do not need to come to the height of resting on the back of your pelvis.

Power It Up
Hold a body bar.

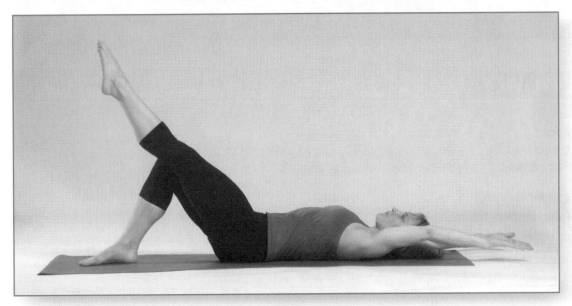

Starting Position: Arms overhead, left leg extended

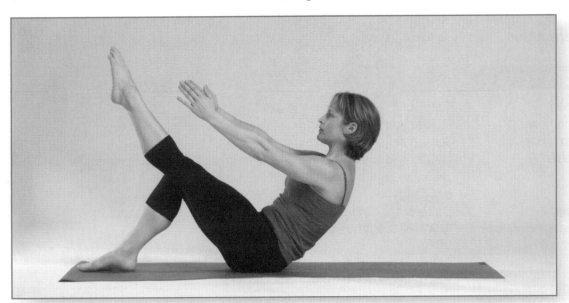

Action: Curl up

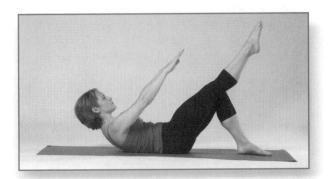

Power It Down: Smaller curl up

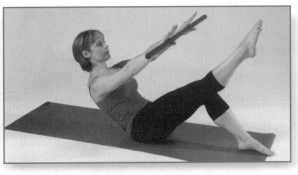

Power It Up: Curl up with Body Bar

Teaser II

Level	Advanced
Purpose	Abdominal strengthening
Prerequisites	Teaser I, page 140; Legs Lower and Lift, 138
Enhancement	Holding the Legs Up, page 90

THE EXERCISES

Starting Position Balance on your tailbone with your legs lifted at a 45 degree angle and your arms parallel to your legs.

Action Inhale as you lower your legs down about 6 inches. Exhale and return your legs to the starting position. There should be no movement at all in your upper body.

Repetitions Perform 4 times.

BODY CHECK

Head Keep your head and neck relaxed.

Shoulders Engage your lats to keep your shoulders pressed down.

Arms/Hands Get the sense of lengthening out through your arms and hands at all times.

Pelvis Initiate and direct the movement from your core. Your abdominals should be deeply engaged throughout the exercise. Do not rock forward or backward on your tailbone.

Legs Contract your buttocks and inner thigh muscles to control the movement.

Feet Your feet should be gently pointed.

You Are Doing It Correctly if you are not using momentum or "flinging" your legs to return to the starting position.

VARIATIONS

Power It Down Hold the starting position for a count of ten.

Power It Up Perform a greater range of motion. Hold a Magic Ring between your legs with your arms reaching overhead.

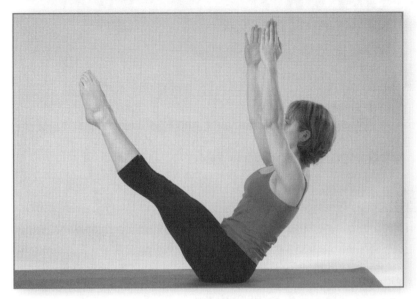

Starting Position: Balance on pelvis

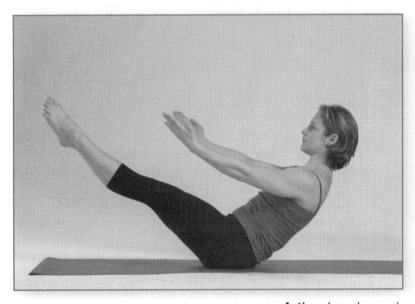

Action: Legs lowered

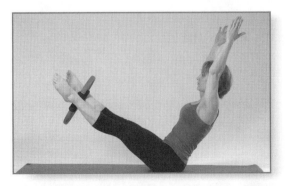

Power It Up: Legs lifted with Magic Ring

Leg Circles

Level	Beginner
Purpose	Pelvic and spine stabilization and improved range of motion of the hip joint
Prerequisite	Straight Leg Stretch, page 128
Enhancement	Hamstring Flexibility, page 84

THE EXERCISES

Starting Position   Lie on your back, arms along your sides, palms down. Bring your **right** leg up so that it is perpendicular to your body.

Action   Inhale as you begin to circle your leg about 2 inches in diameter (a *very small and slow circle)*. Exhale as you complete the circle.

Repetitions   Perform 5 times in one direction, then 5 in the other.

BODY CHECK

Head	Be sure you keep your neck long.
Shoulders	Engage your lats to keep your shoulders down.
Arms/Hands	Reach long through your fingers.
Pelvis	Do not allow your pelvis to move at all. You need to keep your hips completely still and level. As you circle your **right** leg you will feel a tendency to lift your **left** hip up. Tighten your abdominals strongly. Use the image of a block of cement preventing your ribs, spine, and pelvis from any movement whatsoever. This exercise is all about stabilizing.
Legs	Contract the sides of your buttocks and upper legs to turn your leg out.
Feet	Point your feet.

You Are Doing It Correctly if you feel a burning sensation in your abdominals (which means they are fully engaged). This is a particularly difficult exercise to do correctly. Take your time. Go slow.

VARIATIONS

Power It Down   Bend the knee of the leg you are not circling.

Power It Up   Use ankle weights.

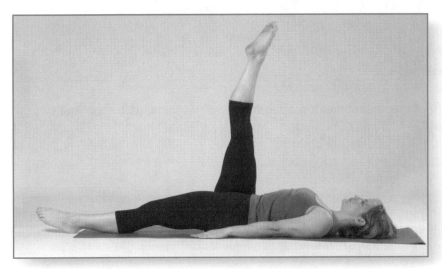

Starting Position: Right leg raised

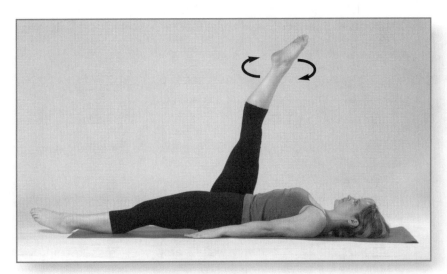

Action: Leg circles

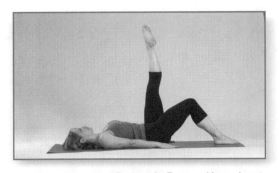

Power It Down: Knee bent

Crisscross

Level	Advanced
Purpose	Strengthen the abdominals with a focus on the obliques
Prerequisites	Pelvic Stabilization, page 42; Single Knee Stretch, page 124; Double Leg Extension, page 126
Enhancement	Holding the Head Up, page 68

THE EXERCISES

Starting Position	Lie on your back with your knees bent and hands behind your head. Lift your head off the floor.
Action	Extend your **left** leg as you twist your torso to the **right**. Then switch to bring your **left** knee into your chest and twist your upper body to the **left** as you straighten your **right** leg. Inhale for one set (right and left), and then exhale for the next.
Repetitions	Perform 10 sets (right and left count as 1 set).

BODY CHECK

Head	Your chin should stay down. Be sure you are not pulling on your head with your hands.
Shoulders	Shoulders should stay down and relaxed.
Arms/Hands	Your fingers should lightly touch the back of your head. Do not allow your elbows to cross over your chest. The twist should begin at your torso and bring your elbows along for the ride.
Pelvis	Stabilize. Imagine a heavy weight atop your torso keeping you nailed to the floor. Do not allow your pelvis to lift as you twist. Keep the **right** side of your back pressed into the floor as you rotate to the **left**, and the **left** side pressed down as you twist to the **right**.
Legs	Lengthen out of the hip joints.
Feet	Gently point your feet.

You Are Doing It Correctly if there is total stabilization with no rocking from side to side.

VARIATIONS

Power It Down	Keep your knees bent throughout.
Power It Down	Add ankle weights to increase difficulty.

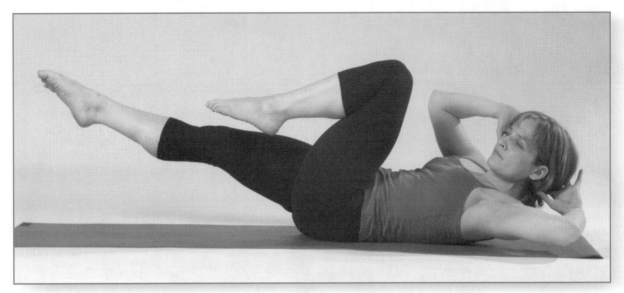

Action: Left knee into chest, right leg extended

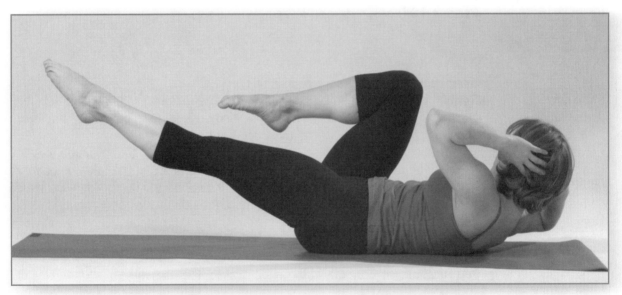

Action: Right knee into chest, left leg extended

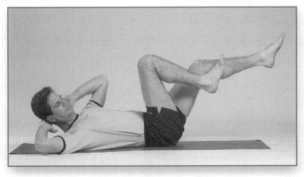

Power It Down: Knees bent

Scissors

Level	Advanced
Purpose	Strengthens the abdominals with a focus on the obliques
Prerequisite	Straight Leg Stretch, page 128
Enhancement	Hamstring Flexibility, page 84

THE EXERCISES

Starting Position	Lie on your back with both legs straight up in the air and your hands behind your head. Lift your head up and keep it there.
Action	Exhale and lower your **right** leg and twist your body to the **left**. Then switch. Breathe in for one set of right and left, and breathe out for the next set.
Repetitions	Perform 10 times (right and left count as 1 set).

BODY CHECK

Head	Keep your head and neck free of tension.
Shoulders	Remind yourself to keep pressing your shoulders down.
Arms/Hands	Do not move your elbows across your body. Keep your elbows back. They should move *as a result of* the twist occurring in your spine.
Pelvis	Imagine your pelvis as a block of cement; do not allow it to move side to side as you twist. As you twist to the **right** focus on contracting the **left** side of your abdominals and keeping the **left** side of your back on the floor. When you twist to the **left** deepen the contraction on the **right** side of your abdominals.
Legs	Turn your legs out from the hip.
Feet	Point your feet.

You Are Doing It Correctly if the work is all in the abdominals *and* the rest of your body is relaxed.

VARIATIONS

Power It Down	Keep your knees bent.
Power It Up	You can make a difficult exercise even harder by using ankle weights.

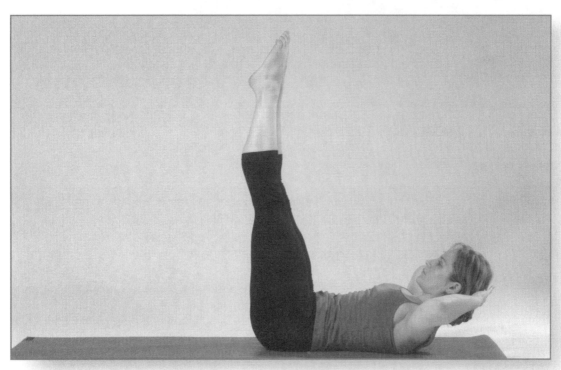

Starting Position: Legs straight up, head raised

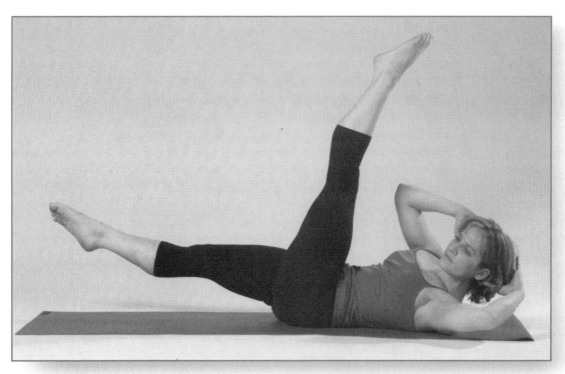

Action: Right leg down, torso twist left

Rollover

Level — Advanced
Purpose — Strengthen the abdominals with an emphasis on the lower fibers
Prerequisite — 90/90, page 130

THE EXERCISES

Starting Position — Lie on your back, arms along your sides, palms down. Bring both legs straight up, perpendicular to your body.

Action — Inhale as you reach through your legs and lift your hips off the mat until your weight is resting on your shoulder blades. Bring your legs over your body until they are parallel to the floor. Exhale and roll down one vertebra at a time until your legs are again perpendicular to your body.

Repetitions — Repeat 5 times.

BODY CHECK

Head — Your neck should be lengthened. (It's important to keep your form correct; see Head Alignment, page 52.)
Shoulders — Keep your shoulders down.
Arms/Hands — Press your palms down into the floor to assist.
Pelvis — Lift your legs up smoothly. Squeeze your buttocks to assist in lifting your legs.
Legs — Your legs should be in the Pilates stance.
Feet — Gently point your feet.

You Are Doing It Correctly if you are moving with control *and* not hurling your legs over your head or letting them fall down quickly when you return.

VARIATIONS

Power It Down — Lift your legs straight up in the air so your pelvis comes off the floor 1 to 2 inches.
Power It Up — Use ankle weights.

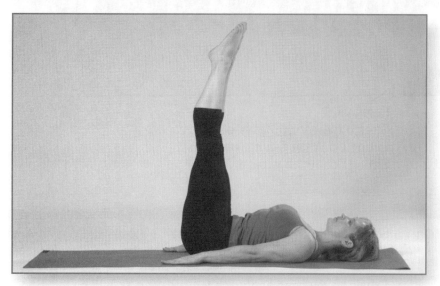

Starting Position: Legs straight up, arms at sides

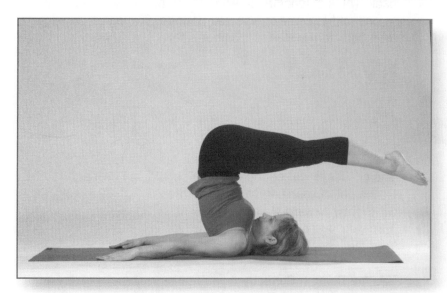

Action: Legs parallel to floor

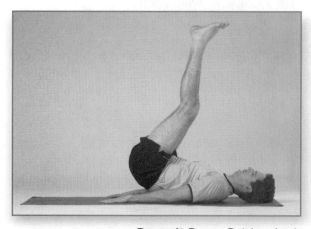

Power It Down: Pelvis raised

Spine Stretch

AT A GLANCE

Level   Beginner
Purpose   Stretch the hamstrings and lower back
Prerequisite   Lifting Up While Sitting, page 56
Enhancement   Sitting Comfortably, page 74

THE EXERCISES

Starting Position   Sit with your legs spread apart about 12 inches and your torso slightly forward of your pelvis. Your arms should be bent and next to your waist.

Action   Exhale as you bend and reach forward. This should be initiated from your lower back. Think of reaching forward as you now inhale and lift your arms and torso as one unit to come to a seated position. Circle your arms out to the side, and then back to the starting position.

Repetitions   Perform 3 times.

BODY CHECK

Head   Keep your head and neck light and free of tension.
Shoulders   The challenge will be to keep your shoulders down and relaxed.
Arms/Hands   Reach out of your fingers in all positions.
Pelvis   Sit slightly forward of your pelvis.
Legs   Turn your legs out from your hips.
Feet   Your feet should be relaxed.

You Are Doing It Correctly if you feel as if someone is trying to pull your arms out of their shoulder sockets through every phase of this exercise *and* your back stays long and lengthened.

VARIATIONS

Power It Down   Find a comfortable seated position. You can keep your knees bent or sit cross-legged.

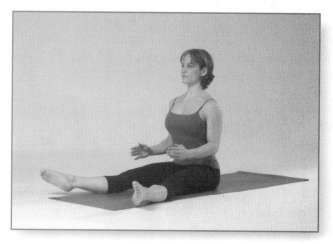

Starting Position: Arms bent at waist

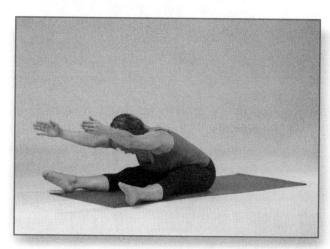

Action 1: Arms straight, bend forward

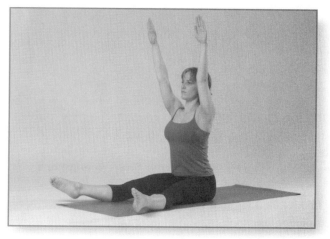

Action 2: Arms up, spine lengthened

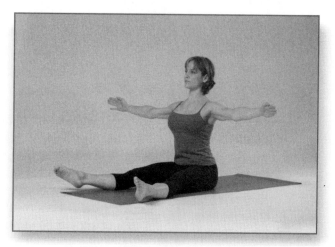

Action 3: Arms out to sides

Seated Twist

Level	Beginner
Purpose	Improve the flexibility of the spine in rotation
Prerequisite	Lifting Up While Sitting, page 56
Enhancements	Sitting Comfortably, page 74; Rotation, page 66; Shoulders Up and Down, page 78

THE EXERCISES

Starting Position	Sit with your legs spread apart comfortably (do not go to your maximum). Hold a Magic Ring* out in front of you.
Action	Exhale and turn your torso to the **right**. Inhale as you come back to the center. Then turn to the **left**.
Repetitions	Perform 3 sets (right and then left count as 1 set).

BODY CHECK

Head	Think of lengthening out of the top of your head.
Shoulders	The challenge will be to keep your shoulders down and relaxed.
Arms/Hands	Press lightly on the Magic Ring.
Pelvis	Sit slightly forward of your pelvis throughout. At the same time, remember to lengthen out of your waist.
Legs	Contract the sides of your buttocks to turn your legs out.
Feet	Your feet should be gently pointed.

You Are Doing It Correctly if you keep your shoulders down.

VARIATIONS

Power It Down	Find a comfortable seated position. You may keep your knees bent, or sit cross-legged.

*If you do not have a Magic Ring, you can use a stretched out towel or simply open your arms out to the side and hold them in this position.

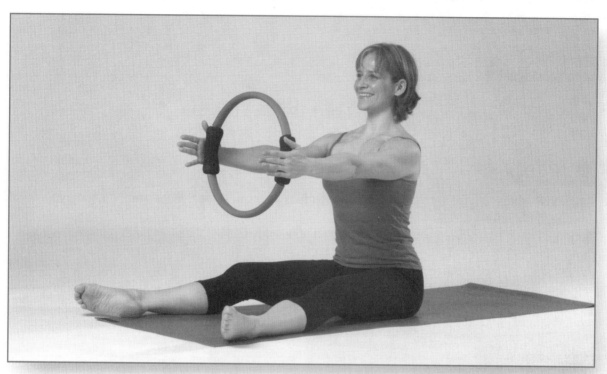

Starting Position: Legs spread holding Magic Ring

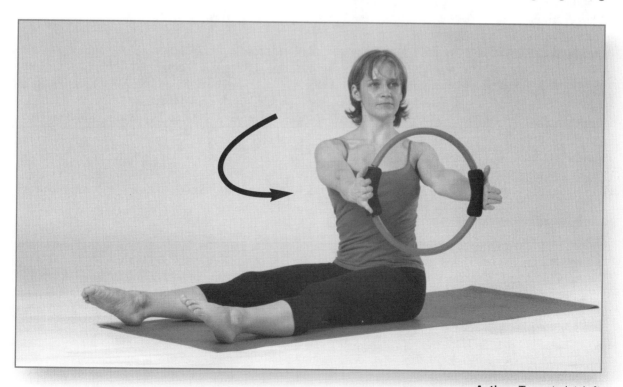

Action: Torso twist left

Rolling Like a Ball

Level	Intermediate
Purpose	Improve flexibility of the spine, whole body coordination, and balance
Enhancement	Rolling, page 98

THE EXERCISES

Starting Position	Sit with your knees pulled into your chest and your hands hugging your legs.
Action	Keep your head down and your body tucked together tightly. Inhale as you roll down and exhale as you roll back up. This is one exercise where you will want to use momentum.
Repetitions	Perform 5 times.

BODY CHECK

Head	Drop your head and nose towards your knees.
Shoulders	Relax your shoulders.
Arms/Hands	Your arms will have a tendency to move away from your legs; try not to let this happen.
Pelvis/Spine	Maintain a fully rounded position throughout. Avoid pounding onto your vertebrae as you roll down; the movement should be even and light. Stay within a small range of motion if needed. Roll down only so far that you will still be able to return to the starting position easily and smoothly.
Legs	Try not to let your legs move away from your body as you roll up. Keep the fully tucked position.
Feet	Keep your feet relaxed.

You Are Doing It Correctly if you keep your shoulders down *and* you're having fun.

VARIATIONS

Power It Down	If you find this exercise difficult, or want to achieve a greater range of motion, take a look at Rolling, page 98, in Chapter 6: *The Secrets to Good Pilates Technique.*

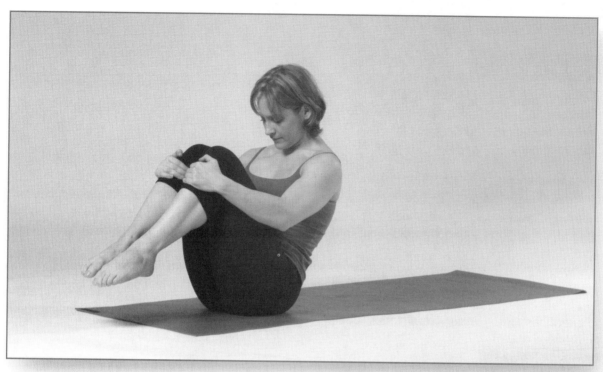

Starting Position: Knees to chest, head down

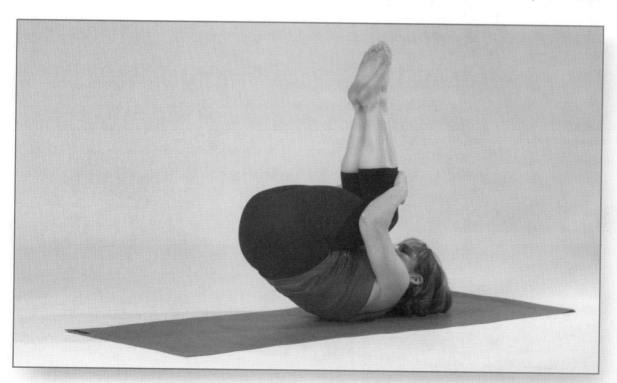

Action: Roll down

Roll Down

Level	Intermediate
Purpose	Strengthen the abdominals and hip flexors
Prerequisite	Roll Up, page 122
Enhancement	Pelvic Tilt, page 70

THE EXERCISES

Starting Position	Sit with your legs and arms extended straight out in front of you. (If this is uncomfortable, sit in a cross-legged or diamond shape position).
Action	Inhale as you tuck your pelvis under and roll **down**. Then exhale and roll back **up** to the starting position.
Repetitions	Perform 4 times.

BODY CHECK

Head	Scan for any tension in your head and neck and release it.
Shoulders	You will feel a tendency to hunch up your shoulders. Counteract this by engaging your lats.
Arms/Hands	Keep reaching with your arms.
Pelvis	Roll down only so far that you will still be able to return to the starting position easily and smoothly. Tightly contract your abdominals to avoid jerking movements or using momentum.
Legs	Turn your legs out from your hips.
Feet	Your feet should be slightly pointed.

You Are Doing It Correctly if the lowering and lifting are very smooth.

VARIATIONS

Power It Down	Do a partial roll down (see Midpoint roll down photo on the next page).
Power It Up	Hold a Magic Ring.

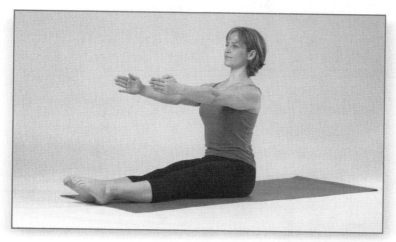

Starting Position: Legs straight, arms extended

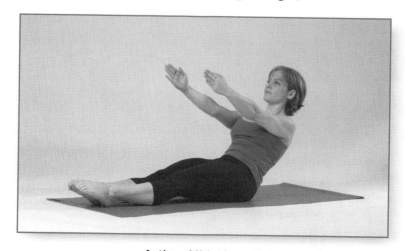

Action: Midpoint roll down, arms extended

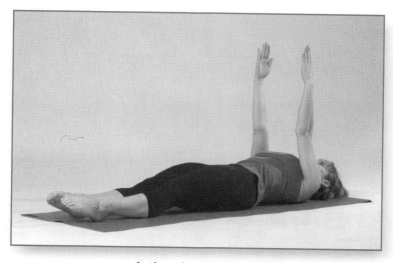

Action: Complete roll down, arms extended

Reverse Hold

AT A GLANCE

Level	Intermediate
Purpose	Strengthen the entire body

THE EXERCISES

Starting Position   Sit in an upright position with your legs straight and your hands* on the floor directly under your shoulders with your fingers pointing towards your buttocks.

Action   Exhale as you lift your body up in the air so you are supported just by your feet and your hands. Inhale and lower down.

Repetitions   Perform 8 times.

BODY CHECK

Head   Your head should be a continuation of your spine, neither drooping down nor hanging back.

Shoulders   Press into your hands to keep your shoulders down and your chest up.

Arms/Hands   Check for correct hand placement, directly under your shoulders.

Pelvis   Engage the core strongly.

Legs   Think of lengthening through your legs.

Feet   Press into your heels for support.

You Are Doing It Correctly if you use your abdominals to keep your body lifted so the middle of your torso is not sagging.

VARIATIONS

Power It Down   Sit with your knees bent and lift your buttocks off the floor so you come into a "tabletop" position.

* Or on your knuckles.

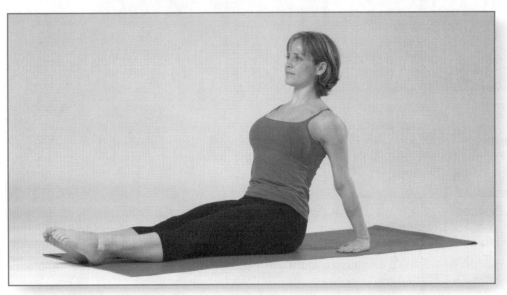

Starting Position: Legs straight, hands on floor

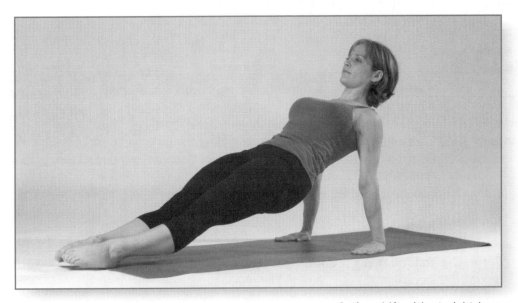

Action: Lift with straight legs

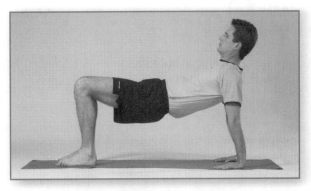

Power It Down: Lift with bent knees

Leg Pull Front

AT A GLANCE

Level	Advanced
Purpose	Strengthens the entire body
Prerequisite	Reverse Hold, page 160

THE EXERCISES

Starting Position Sit in an upright position, your hands* on the floor directly under your shoulders. Lift your body up in the air so just your hands and feet support you.

Action Exhale as you lift your **right** leg. Inhale as you lower it. Your torso should stay lifted throughout.

Repetitions Perform 8 times with your **right** leg, then 8 times with your **left**. Do all the repetitions for one leg before moving on to the other.

BODY CHECK

Head Your head should be a continuation of your spine, neither on your chest nor hanging back.

Shoulders Keep your shoulders down and your chest lifted.

Arms/Hands Check for correct hand placement, directly under your shoulders.

Pelvis Do not allow your pelvis or hips to move. Counteract the tendency to lower your hips as you lift your leg.

Legs Feel as if your leg is being lengthened as you lift and lower it. Use the Pilates Stance.

Feet Press into your heels for support.

You Are Doing It Correctly if you do not allow your hips to lower as you lift your leg.

VARIATIONS

Power It Down Come to the Reverse Hold position and hold for a count of 10.

Power It Up Use ankle weights.

*You can also be on your knuckles.

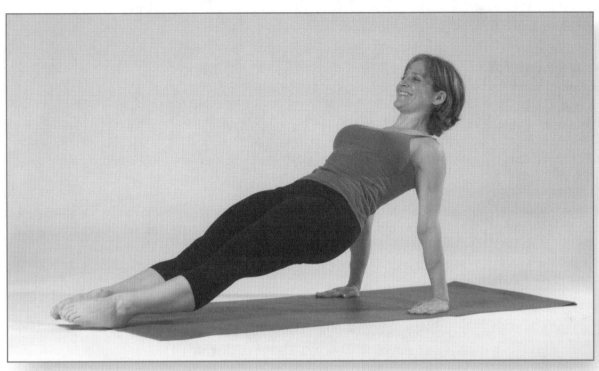

Starting Position: Reverse Hold position

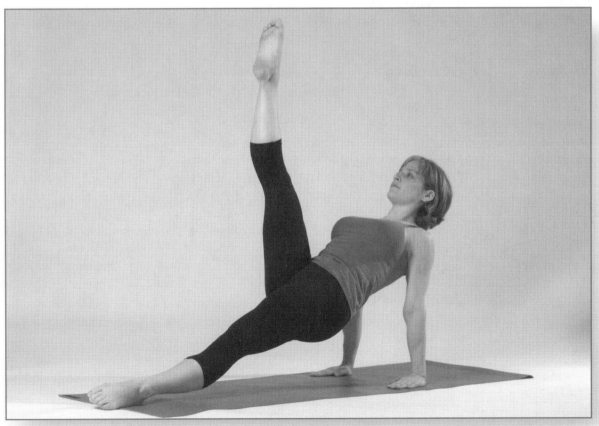

Action: Reverse Hold with right leg raised

Side Leg Series

Level	Beginner
Purpose	Tone the entire leg
Prerequisite	Turning Out From the Hip, page 54
Enhancements	Hamstring Flexibility, page 84; Inner Thigh Flexibility, page 86

THE EXERCISES

Starting Position

Lie on your **left** side with your head supported by your **left** hand.* Bring both legs *slightly* in front of you and curl your right toes under so they are in standing position. Your **right** leg should be extended long and in the Pilates Stance.

Action

1. Up and down. Flex your **right** foot and turn your leg out from your hip. Exhale as you lift your leg. Point your foot and lower your leg as you exhale.
2. Front and back. Flex your **right** foot. Exhale as you bring your leg forward. Inhale, point your foot and bring your leg back past the middle to extend in back of you.
3. Small circles. Point your **right** foot with your leg in the Pilates Stance. Lift it up a few inches away from your **left** leg and make small circles in one direction. Then circle in the other direction.

Repetitions

Do all the exercises on one side before switching to the other side. Perform each movement 10 times (up and down, or forward and back, is one movement).

BODY CHECK

Head	Keep your head and neck light and free of tension.
Shoulders	Pay attention to how you are supporting your upper body. Do not sag into your shoulders. Press into your forearm on the floor to keep your shoulders from hunching up.
Arms/Hands	One hand should support your head while the other is on the floor in front of you.
Pelvis/Spine	Engage your core throughout to maintain spinal and pelvic stabilization. Neither your upper body nor your hips should move at all. Your leg should be the lone moving part.
Legs	Lengthen, lengthen, lengthen. Feel as if your leg is continually being pulled out of your hip socket.
Feet	See the instructions for each exercise.

VARIATIONS

You Are Doing It Correctly if you feel the work in your abdominals *as well as* in the back and sides of your legs. In Up and Down (Action 1) you should feel a stretch in your inner thighs.
You Are Doing It Incorrectly if there is any tension along the front of your thigh or your groin area.

Power It Up

Use ankle weights.
*Alternatively, you can allow your head to rest on your arm, or put a rolled up towel under your head for support.

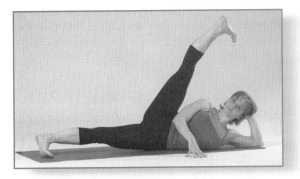

Action 1: Right leg up, foot flexed

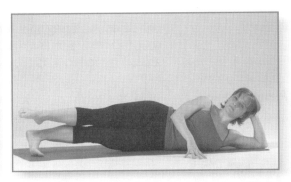

Action 1: Right leg down, foot pointed

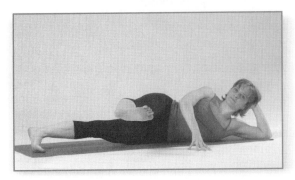

Action 2: Right leg forward, foot flexed

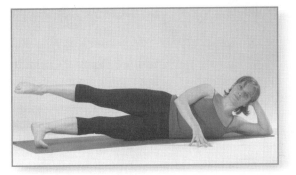

Action 2: Right leg backward, foot pointed

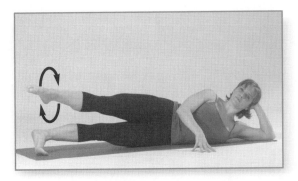

Action 3: Right leg circles, foot pointed

Side Stretch

Level   Beginner
Purpose   Stretch the lats, waist, and sides of the hips

THE EXERCISES

Starting Position   Sit with your **right** knee bent in front of your body and your **left** leg bent in back, forming a "Z." Place your **right** hand on the floor next to your **right** side.

Action   Exhale as you bring your **left** arm overhead and lift your hips off the floor. Turn your head more to the **right** to look past your **left** hand. (If your knees or back are uncomfortable, do not do this exercise).

Repetitions   Hold the stretch for a slow count of 10. Keep breathing as you hold the position. With each exhalation deepen into the stretch. Continue by performing the stretch on the other side.

BODY CHECK

Head   Imagine your head lightly floating above your spine.
Shoulders   Do not allow your shoulders to hunch up.

You Are Doing It Correctly if you feel a stretch from under your armpit down to the side of your waist and hip.

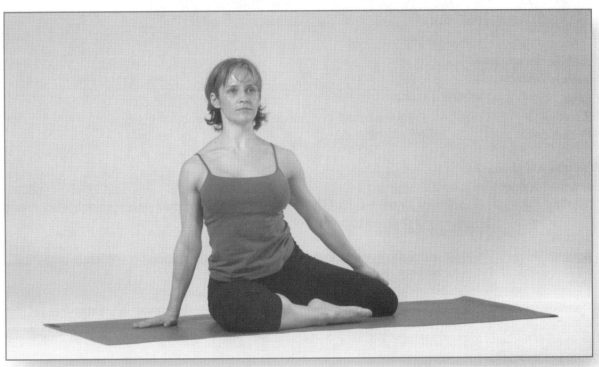

Starting Position: Right knee bent in front

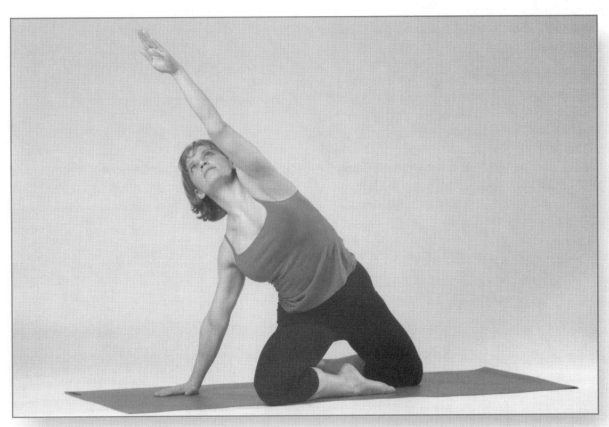

Action: Left arm overhead, hips raised

Mermaid

Level	Advanced
Purpose	Strengthen the upper body and stretch the waist and side of the hips
Prerequisite	Side Stretch, page 166

THE EXERCISES

Starting Position	Lie on your **right** side. Lift up and support your body with your **right** hand* and the side of your **right** foot.
Action	Lift your **left** arm so it is next to your ear and extended completely straight. (If you feel any pain in your wrist or shoulder, stop).
Repetitions	Hold the stretch for a slow count of 10. Don't hold your breath. Repeat the stretch on the other side.

BODY CHECK

Head	Think of your head as a continuation of your spine.
Shoulders	Do not allow the shoulder of your supporting arm to hunch up.
Arms/Hands	Your flat hand or knuckles should be on the floor directly under your shoulder joint. The extended arm should be next to your ear and not out in front. Reach through your fingertips as you stretch.
Waist/Pelvis	Engage your abdominals to lift your side away from the floor.
Legs	Lengthen through your legs.
Feet	Your feet should be relaxed.

You Are Doing It Correctly if you feel a stretch from under your left armpit and down along the left side of your torso, your hips remain lifted so that you form a straight line, *and* you remember to breathe.

*You can also be on your knuckles.

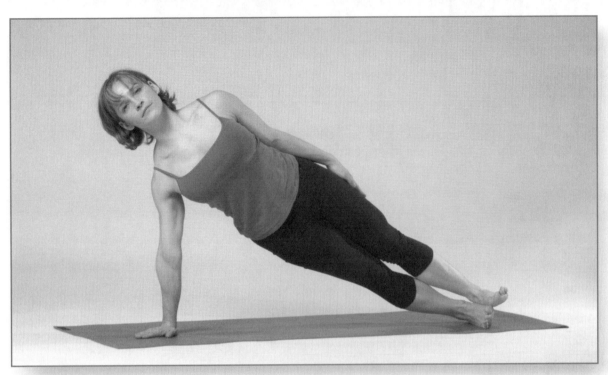

Starting Position: Raised on right arm and right foot

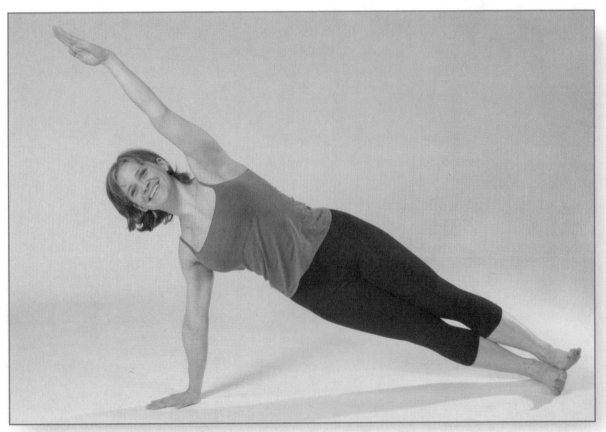

Action: Left arm extended, head turned right

Push-Up Hold

Level	Beginner
Purpose	Strengthen the upper body and the core
Prerequisites	Hand and Finger Positioning, page 58
Enhancement	Shoulders Together and Apart, page 82

THE EXERCISES

Starting Position   Assume the Push-Up position. You should be on your toes with your hands *directly* under your shoulders.

Action   Maintain this position. Keep breathing normally.

Repetitions   Hold for a slow count of 10.

BODY CHECK

Head   Lengthen your head out of your spine. Do not let it hang down.

Shoulders   Bring your shoulders blades apart (see enhancement).

Arms/Hands   Pay close attention to the position of your hands; they should be *directly* under your shoulders. Avoid having them far apart or out in front.

Spine/Pelvis   Watch out for sagging in your mid-section; engage your abdominals and keep them lifted. Try to form a straight line from the top of your head to your toes.

You Are Doing It Correctly if you feel the work occurring in your abdominals *and* you continue to breathe.

VARIATIONS

Power It Down   Support yourself on your *elbows* and toes.

Power It Up   Hold for a slow count of 20.

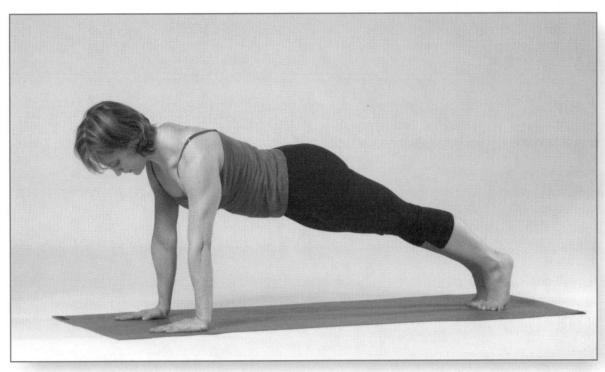

Action: Push-Up position

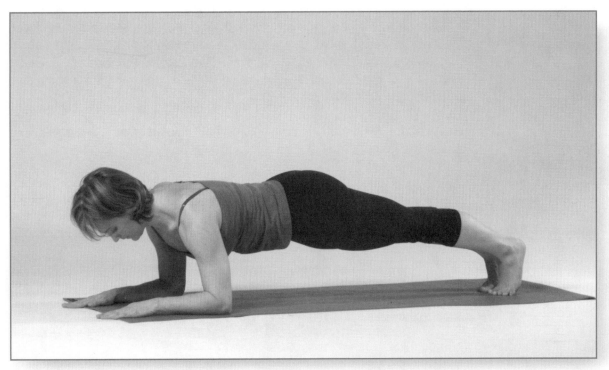

Power It Down: Elbow Push-Up position

Leg Pull Back

Level	Advanced
Purpose	All over body strengthening with emphasis on the upper body and core
Prerequisite	Push-Up Hold, page 170
Enhancement	Shoulders Together and Apart, page 82

THE EXERCISES

Starting Position On your hands and toes in the Push-Up position.

Action Exhale and lift your **left** leg up about 6 inches. Inhale and lower it back down.

Repetitions Perform 8 repetitions with your right leg followed by 8 repetitions with your left leg.

BODY CHECK

Head Maintain good head alignment; do not allow your head to droop down.

Shoulders Make sure your shoulders stay down.

Arms/Hands Be sure that your hands are *directly* under your shoulders. This may be a smaller distance than you are used to and therefore may feel much harder.

Pelvis Do not raise your hips as you lift your **left** leg—your hips should remain level. This exercise is not about how high you can raise your leg but rather about upper body strength and maintaining pelvic and spinal stabilization.

Legs Lengthen your **right** leg out of your hip socket as you lift and lower it.

Feet Gently point your foot as you lift your leg.

You Are Doing It Correctly if your hips do not move as you lift and lower your leg *and* you do not sag in the middle.

VARIATIONS

Power It Down Go onto your hands and knees (see 4 Point Leg Series). Extend your **right** leg in back of you, and lift and lower the leg.

Power It Up Ankle weights can be added.

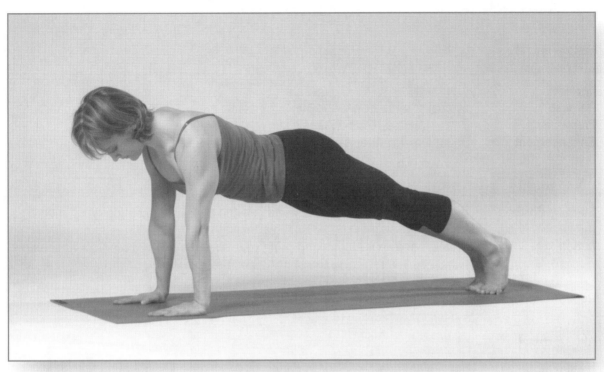

Starting Position: Push-Up position

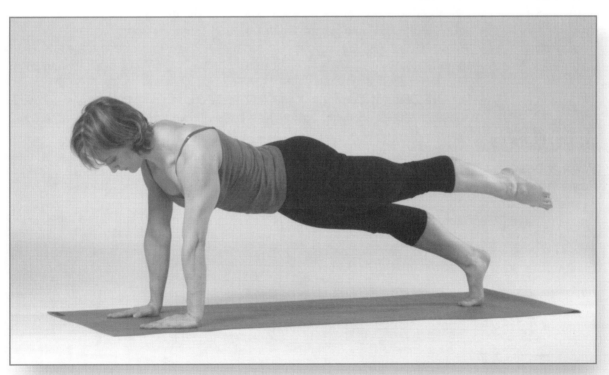

Action: Left leg lift

Push-Ups

Level	Intermediate
Purpose	Strengthen the upper body and the core
Prerequisite	Push-Up Hold, page 170
Enhancement	Shoulders Together and Apart, page 82

THE EXERCISES

Starting Position Begin on your toes with your hands on the floor *directly* under your shoulders.

Action Inhale, bend your elbows and bring your chest as close to the floor as possible. Exhale as you return to the starting position.

Repetitions Perform 10 times.

BODY CHECK

Head Sense your head as a continuation of your spine. Do not allow it to droop.

Shoulders Keep your shoulders down.

Arms/Hands Pay close attention to the position of your hands; they should be *directly* under your shoulders. Avoid having them far apart or out in front.

Spine/Pelvis Watch out for sagging in your mid-section; engage your abdominals and keep them lifted. Try to form a straight line from the top of your head to your toes.

You Are Doing It Correctly if you feel the work in your abdominals *and* your shoulder blades are lying flat on your back *and* you continue to breathe.

VARIATIONS

Power It Down Perform the exercise on your hands and knees.

Power It Up Perform 20 repetitions.

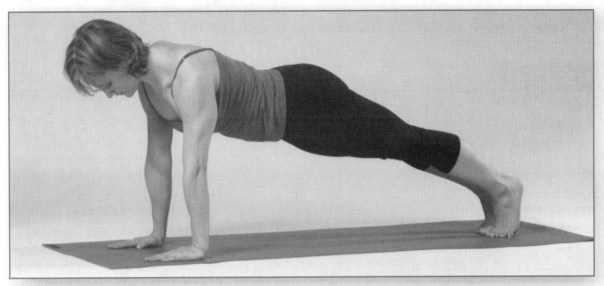

Starting Position: Push-Up position

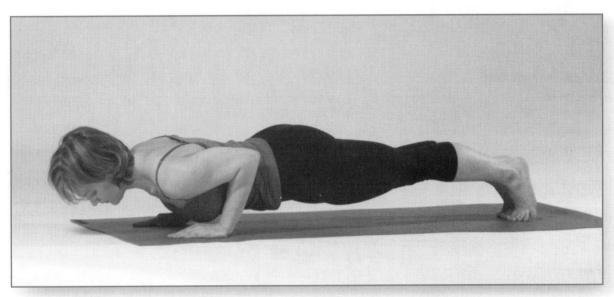

Action: Elbows bent, chest to floor

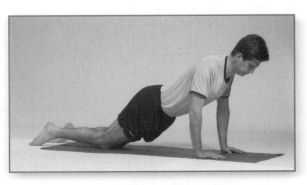

Power It Down: Knee push-ups

4 Points

AT A GLANCE

Level   Beginner
Purpose   Strengthen all the muscles of your back and posterior leg; improve balance
Enhancement   Preparing for Back Work II, page 94

THE EXERCISES

Starting Position   The 4 points position is on your hands* and knees.

Action   As you exhale reach your **right** arm and **left** leg up from the floor and away from you. Your arm should reach forward while the opposite leg extends back. Inhale and return to the starting position. Change to the **left** arm and **right** leg.

Repetitions   Perform 6 alternating sets (**right** arm, **left** leg *and* **left** arm, **right** leg count as 1 set).

BODY CHECK

Head/Neck   Pretend someone is standing in front of you and pulling gently on your neck to lengthen it.

Shoulders   Keep your shoulders down on your back.

Arms/Hands   Place your hands (or knuckles) directly under your shoulders. Lengthen your arm as you lift.

Waist/Pelvis   Your goal is to keep your hips stable and parallel (or square) to the floor. Concentrate on keeping your **right** hip down when you lift your **right** leg, and keeping your **left** hip down when you lift your **left** leg.

Legs   Straighten your leg completely and lengthen it away from you as you lift. Focus more on lengthening your leg rather than lifting it.

Feet   Gently point your foot as you extend your leg.

You Are Doing It Correctly if there is no shift of your hips when you change arms and legs *and* your hips level.

VARIATIONS

Power It Down   Keep a bend in your arm and leg as you lift.
Power It Up   Use ankle and wrist weights.

*You can also be on your knuckles, or even supported on your forearms.

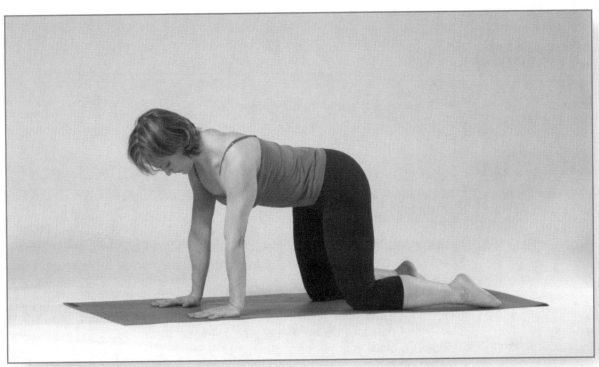

Starting Position: On hands and knees

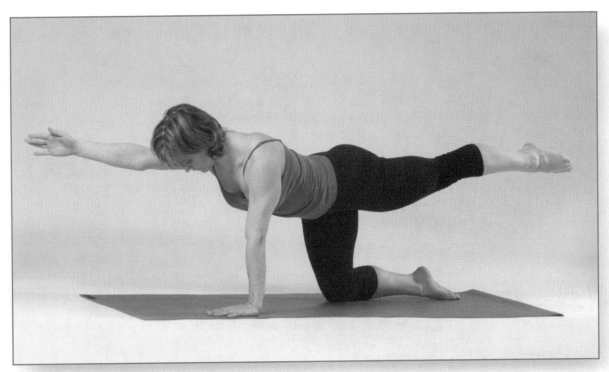

Action: Right arm forward, left leg back

4 Points Leg Series

AT A GLANCE

Level	Beginner
Purpose	Tone the legs and strengthen the core
Prerequisite	4 Points, 176

THE EXERCISES

Starting Position
Begin in the 4 points position with your **left** leg long, turned out, and lifted off the floor.

Action

1. Lower and lift. Bring your **right** arm straight ahead and lower your **left** leg so both arm and leg are touching the floor. Exhale as you lift your **right** arm and **left** leg simultaneously. Inhale as you lower them.

2. Knee to chest. Inhale as you bring your **left** knee in towards your chest, and exhale as you extend it backward so that it is once again lifted off the floor to the starting position. Do not swing your leg or arch your back.

3. Side lift. Move your hands to the **right**. Swing your **left** leg around to the **left** side and off the floor. From here, inhale as you lower your **left** leg, and exhale as you lift it.

Repetitions
Perform 6 times with your right leg, then 6 times with the left.

BODY CHECK

Head	Keep your head lengthened out of your spine and avoid letting it fall down.
Shoulders	Remember to keep your shoulder blades down.
Arms/Hands	Place your hands (or knuckles) directly under your shoulders.
Waist/Pelvis	Your goal is to not let your hips move—keep your pelvis parallel to the floor. You will feel inclined to raise your **right** hip as you lift your **right** leg, and vice versa. Focus on your core: keep your abdominals lifted throughout.
Legs	Keep lengthening out of your leg.
Feet	Gently point your foot.

You Are Doing It Correctly if your pelvis remains square to the floor *and* you continually feel as if someone is trying to pull your leg out of its socket.

VARIATIONS

Power It Down	Perform actions 1 and 2 with a slight bend in your knee throughout the movement. Do not perform action 3.
Power It Up	Strap on ankle weights.

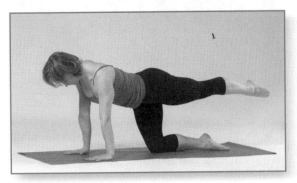

Starting Position: 4 points position, left leg raised

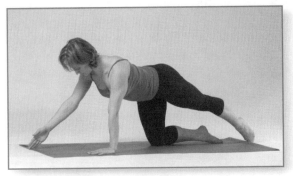

Action 1: Right arm and left leg down

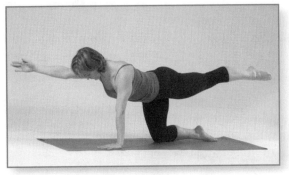

Action 1: Right arm and left leg lift

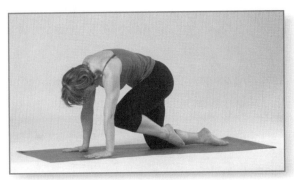

Action 2: Left leg tuck

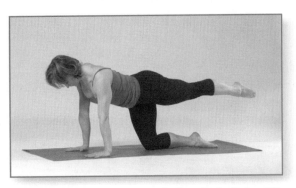

Action 2: Left leg lift

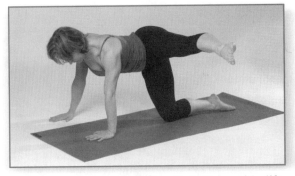

Action 3: Left leg side lift

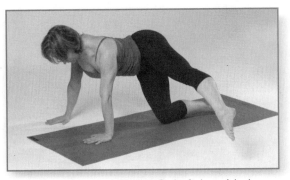

Action 3: Left leg side lower

Swan

Level   Beginner
Purpose   Increase the flexibility of the spine in extension
Enhancement   Preparing for Back Work I, page 92

THE EXERCISES

Starting Position   Lie on your stomach with your hands* on the floor next to your shoulders.

Action   Inhale as you *slowly* straighten your elbows and lift your upper body away from the floor. Exhale and bend your elbows to return to the starting position. (If you feel any pain, stop).

Repetitions   Hold the stretch for a slow count of 10.

BODY CHECK

Head   Allow your head to lift up in tandem with your spine. Don't drop your head back; lengthen out of the top of your head.

Shoulders   Keep your shoulders down.

Arms/Hands   Place your hands next to your shoulders. Think of lifting from your chest as you straighten your elbows.

Pelvis   Pull your abdominals in as you *inhale.*

Legs   Turn your legs out. Squeeze your buttocks and the upper portion of your inner thigh muscles.

Feet   Your feet should be gently pointed.

You Are Doing It Correctly if you are able to arch your back a little with no pain.

VARIATIONS

Power It Down   Place your forearms on the floor. Lift your head up slightly until you feel your back arching.

* Or knuckles.

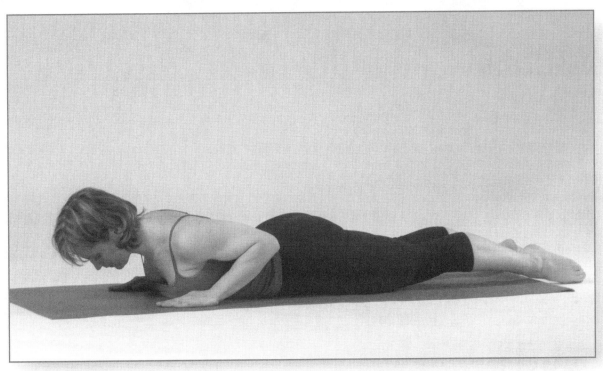

Starting Position: Hands beside shoulders

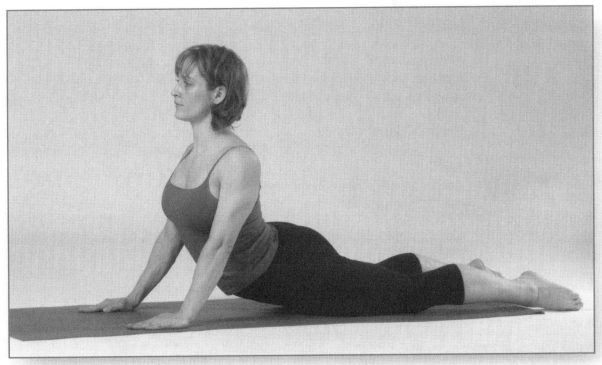

Action: Elbows straight, upper body raised

Flight

Level	Beginner
Purpose	Strengthen the muscles of the back
Prerequisite	Swan, page 180
Enhancement	Preparing for Back Work I, page 92

THE EXERCISES

Starting Position   Lie on your stomach with your arms *directly* out to your sides.

Action   Exhale as you bring your arms down next to your sides and lift your upper body off the floor. Keep pressing the tops of your feet into the floor. Inhale, lower down, and return your arms back out to your sides.

Repetitions   Perform 6 times.

BODY CHECK

Head   Allow your head to raise as you lift your torso. Imagine you are lengthening out of the top of your head.

Shoulders   Engage your lats to lower your shoulders.

Arms/Hands   Bring your arms down to your sides first, and then lift your head.

Pelvis   When you exhale, use the Deep Abdominal Contraction.

Legs   Your legs should be in the Pilates Stance.

Feet   Press the tops of your feet into the floor.

You Are Doing It Correctly if you perform the movement smoothly and slowly *and* feel the right and left sides of your back working equally to lift your head and torso.

VARIATIONS

Power It Up   Bring your arms straight out to the sides (Airplane Arms). Do not move them down by your sides, even a little, as you begin the lift. You should be able to see your hands in your peripheral vision.

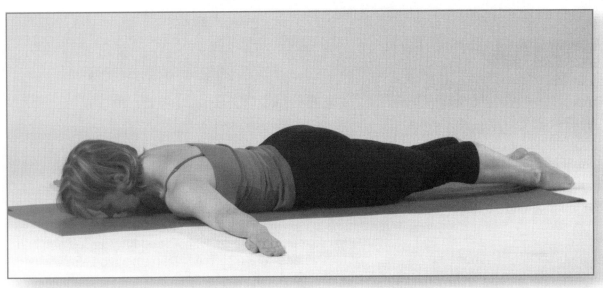

Starting Position: On stomach, arms out

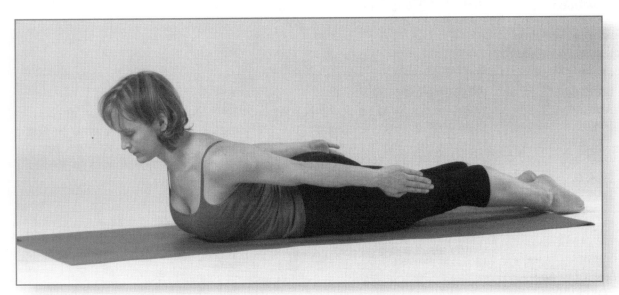

Action: Arms by sides, upper body raised

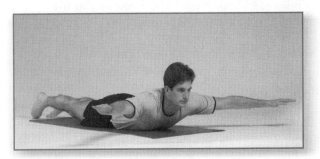

Power It Up: Upper body lift with airplane arms

Opposite Arm and Leg Lift

Level	Beginner
Purpose	Strengthen the back; tone the buttocks and legs
Prerequisite	Flight, page 182;
Enhancement	Preparing for Back Work II, page 94

THE EXERCISES

Starting Position	Lie on your stomach with your arms out in front (like Superman flying).
Action	Inhale and reach through your arms and legs. Exhale and lift your **left** arm and **right** leg off the floor. Inhale and return to the starting position. Exhale and switch, this time lifting your **right** arm and **left** leg.
Repetitions	Perform 10 sets (**right** and **left** count as 1 set).

BODY CHECK

Head	Your head and neck remain free of tension.
Shoulders	Engage your lats.
Arms/Hands	Your palms should be down as you continually lengthen out of your arms.
Pelvis	Even when in a prone position your goal is pelvic stabilization. Keep both hips pressing into the floor. As you lift your **left** leg off the floor you will feel a tendency to raise your **left** hip, and vice versa. Do not allow this to happen.
Legs	Contract the sides of your buttocks to turn your legs out.
Feet	Your feet should be gently pointed.

You Are Doing It Correctly if your pelvis does not shift from side to side as you switch arms and legs *and* you feel that you're being stretched out from head to toe.

VARIATIONS

Power It Down	Keep a bend at your elbow and knee as you lift.
Power It Up	Use wrist and ankle weights.

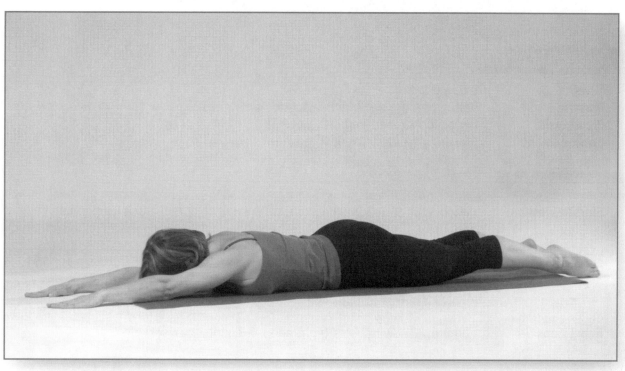

Starting Position: Superman position

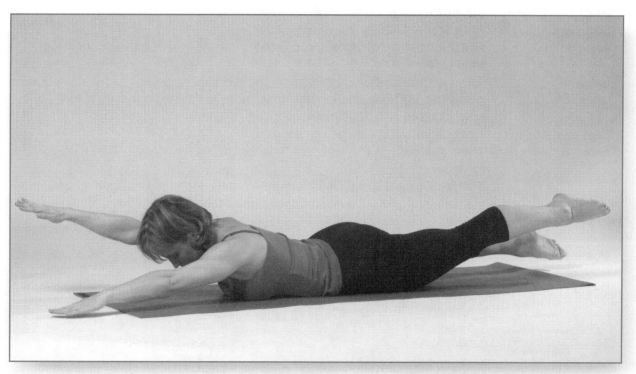

Action: Left arm and right leg raised

Swimming

Level — Intermediate
Purpose — Strengthen the back, gluteals, and hamstrings
Prerequisite — Opposite Arm and Leg Lift, page 184
Enhancement — Preparing for Back Work II, page 94

THE EXERCISES

Starting Position — Lie on your stomach with your arms straight out in front (Superman flying position).

Action — Lift both arms and legs off the floor. Now flutter your arms and legs in opposition (**right** arm and **left** leg will be high at the same time). Alternate as you inhale for 5 sets of **right** and **left**, and then exhale for 5 sets.

Repetitions — Perform 20 "swim" sets (right and left counts as 1 set).

BODY CHECK

Head — Lengthen your head out of your spine.
Shoulders — Keep your shoulders free of tension.
Arms/Hands — Reach through your arms and pretend someone is trying to pull them out of their sockets.
Pelvis — This exercise is about stabilization and elongation. Do not allow your ribs or pelvis to shift from side to side. Your entire torso should remain stable while only your arms and legs move.
Legs — Keep lengthening out through your legs.
Feet — Point your feet.

You Are Doing It Correctly if your pelvis does not shift from side to side *and* you feel as if you're being stretched out from both ends of your body.

VARIATIONS

Power It Down — Make slow movements, alternating your right arm and left leg, then your left arm and right leg.
Power It Up — Use ankle and wrist weights.

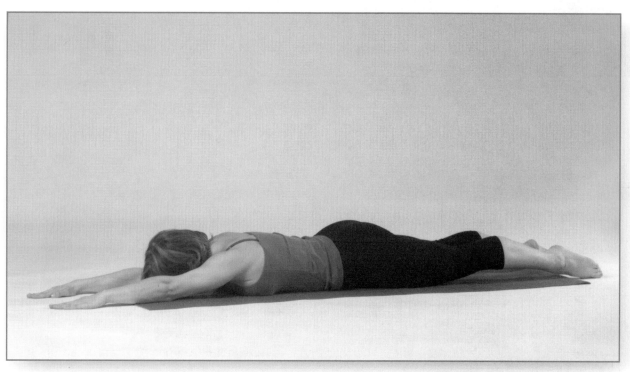

Starting Position: Superman position

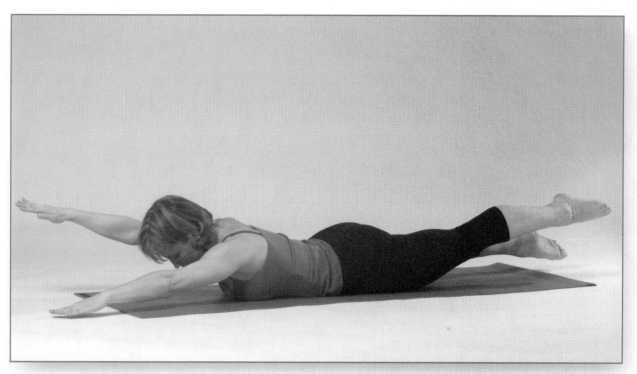

Action: Right arm and left leg flutter

Double Leg Lift

Level	Intermediate
Purpose	Strengthen your back, gluteals, and hamstrings
Prerequisite	Opposite Arm and Leg Lift, page 184
Enhancement	Preparing for Back Work II, page 94

THE EXERCISES

Starting Position	Begin in the Superman Flying position.
Action	Exhale as you lift both legs, and inhale as you lower them back down.
Repetitions	Perform 10 times.

BODY CHECK

Head	Your head and upper body should remain still; do not bob your head up and down.
Shoulders	Use your lat muscles to keep your shoulders down.
Arms/Hands	Keep reaching out through your arms.
Pelvis	Engage your abdominals and press both your hips into the floor.
Legs	Use the Pilates Stance. Try not to let your knees bend as you lift your legs.
Feet	Point your feet.

You Are Doing It Correctly if you lengthen your legs as you lift them *and* your knees do not bend at all.

VARIATIONS

Power It Up	Use ankle weights and double the number of repetitions.

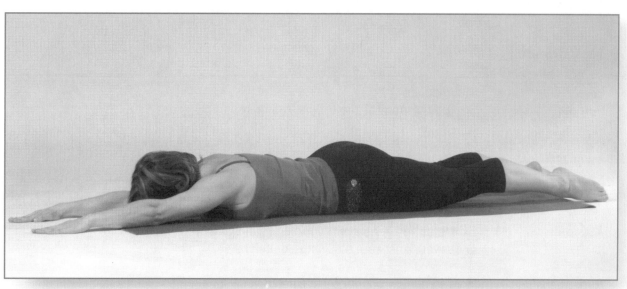

Starting Position: Superman position

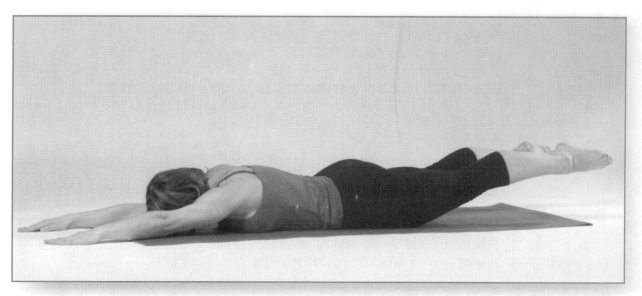

Action: Legs raised

Quad Stretch

Level	Intermediate
Purpose	Stretch the front of the thighs (quadriceps)

THE EXERCISES

Starting Position Prop yourself up on your elbows and bend your **left** knee. *Slowly** reach around to grab somewhere on your lower **left** leg or ankle.

Action Exhale as you gently pull your leg in closer to your buttocks. (If you feel pain under your kneecap, stop immediately).

Repetitions Hold for a slow count of 10. Then switch legs.

BODY CHECK

Head	Keep your neck long; don't allow your head to hang down.
Shoulders	Both of your shoulders should face forward; do not twist or contort your body.
Chest	Keep your chest lifted.
Pelvis	Press both front hipbones into the mat to keep your pelvis level.
Legs	Stop immediately if you feel any cramping about to begin. Stretch that area. Then try to move slowly into the exercise again.
Feet	Relax your feet.

You Are Doing It Correctly if you feel a stretch along the front of your thigh *and* have no pain in your knee.

* Many people begin to cramp in their back, leg, or foot with this exercise. Be sure to move very slowly as you begin. Keep your entire body relaxed, and gently exhale as you reach around to grab your ankle.

Power It Up For more of a stretch lift the knee of the leg you're stretching off the floor.

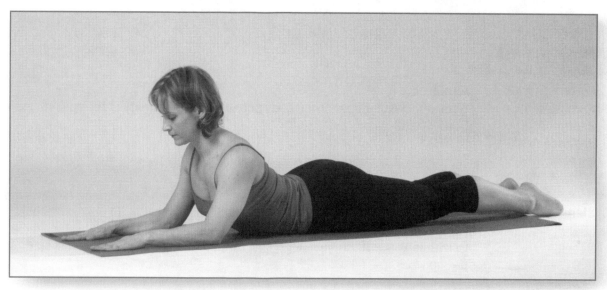

Starting Position: Lying on elbows

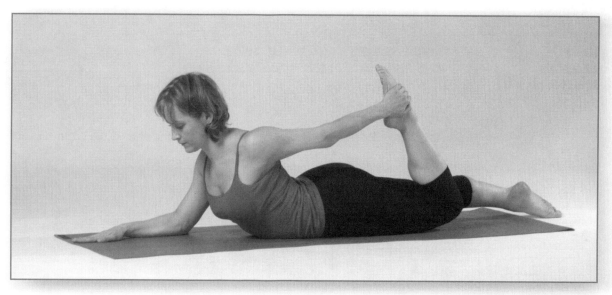

Action: Left leg pull

Rocking

AT A GLANCE

Level	Advanced
Purpose	Stretch the whole front of the body and increase the ability of the spine to arch
Prerequisite	Quad Stretch, page 190 *
Enhancement	Hip Flexor Flexibility, page 88

THE EXERCISES

Starting Position	Lie on your stomach, bend both knees, and reach around to hold both feet.
Action	Inhale as you pull on your legs and raise your chest. Return to the starting position.
Repetitions	Perform 4 times.

BODY CHECK

Head	Your head is a continuation of your spine.
Shoulders	Use your lats to pull your shoulders blades down.
Arms/Hands	Try to keep your elbows in a straight, gently locked position.
Pelvis	Inhale as you *pull in* your abdominals and exhale as you release them.

You Are Doing It Correctly if you feel a stretch along the whole front of your body—arms, torso, and legs—without any pain.

* Always do the previous mat exercise, Quad Stretch, before you do this one.

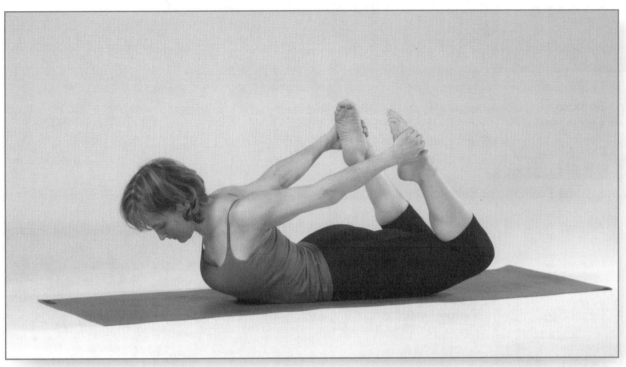

Starting Position: Arms straight, holding feet

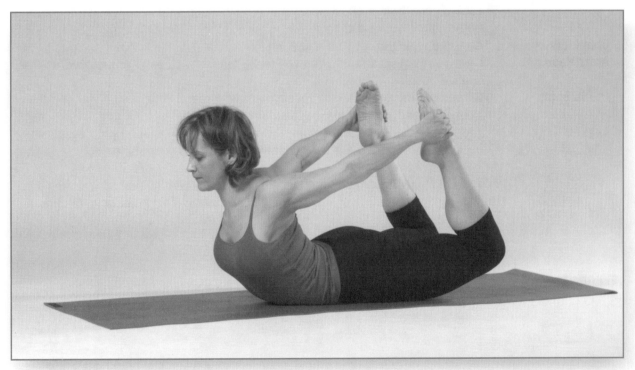

Action: Chest raised

Cat Stretch

Level	Beginner
Purpose	Flexibility of the spine
Enhancement	Pelvic Tilt, page 70

THE EXERCISES

Starting Position Begin on your hands and knees.

Action Exhale and tuck your pelvis under, drop your head, and arch your back (imagine you are a stretching cat) as you try to bring your nose towards your belly button. Inhale as you *slowly* let go of your stomach and then *slowly* reverse the arch. Aim to lift your chest forward and up.

Repetitions Perform 4 times, holding each position for a slow count of 5.

BODY CHECK

Head Move your head down toward your chest as far as it will go as you arch your back. Then lift your chest up as much as you can when you reverse the arch. Do not throw your head back.

Shoulders Avoid hunching up at your shoulders.

Arms/Hands Keep your elbows straight. You will feel a tendency to bend your elbows as you change positions.

Pelvis/Spine Initiate the movements with your breathing. Expand your ribs fully as you take in oxygen, and allow your ribs to soften as you exhale.

Legs Your knees should be slightly apart. Don't shift your weight on your legs or lean backward; the movement should only occur only in your spine.

You Are Doing It Correctly if you are using your breath to expand your ribs and increase the rounding of your spine, *and* exhaling fully to allow your spine to become concave.

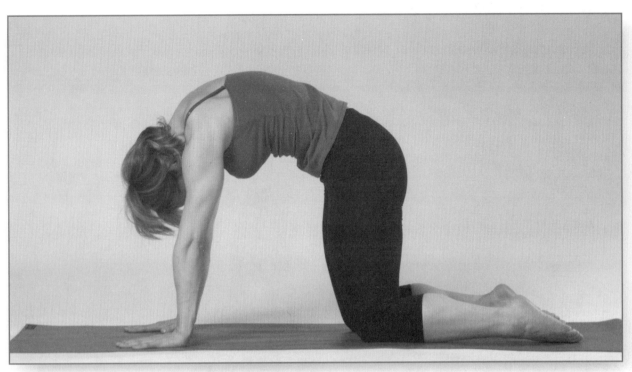

Action: Back Arch

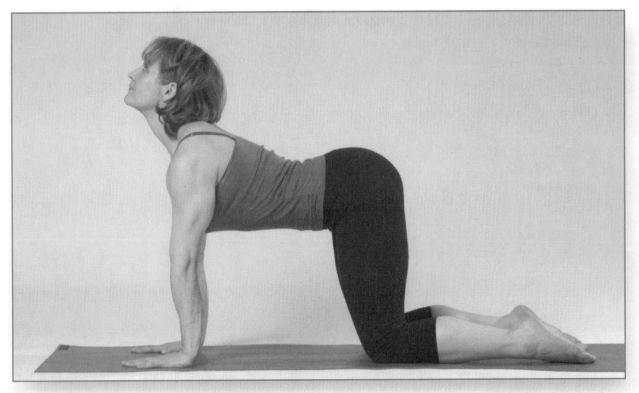

Action: Reverse Arch

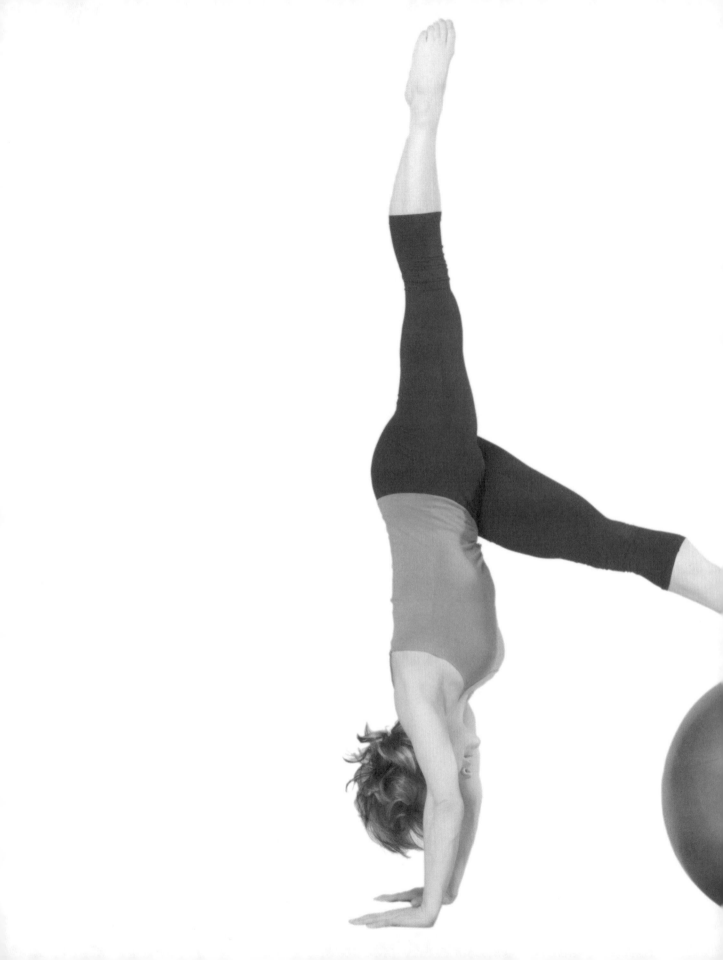

Chapter 9

The Ball Exercises

A Fun Way to Do Pilates

*T*here have been many adaptations of the work of Joseph Pilates over the years, and the stability ball is one of them. Originally used for physical therapy the ball has found its way into sports training. Now a staple of most health clubs, the ball easily lends itself to working on *core stabilization,* the foundation on which the Pilates method is built. Every ball exercise recruits your abdominal and back muscles to create a girdle of strength in your mid-section.

It is impossible to do these exercises without elevating the level of your focus and concentration. You must also intensify the contractions of your deep abdominal musculature or you will find yourself slipping and sliding off the ball. For your efforts you can expect to be greatly rewarded with improved balance and coordination that will carry over into your everyday life, your recreational pastimes, or any athletic endeavor you undertake.

Choosing the Right Ball Exercises

To do the ball exercises correctly you must be able to transfer the principles of stabilization to an unstable surface. With its circular configuration, a ball will roll easily in any direction. So the challenge of stabilization, difficult enough on a stationary floor, is amplified.

Exercises that are listed as appropriate for *All Levels* are generally stretches. It is extremely pleasant to use the ball as you strive to improve your flexibility. You will enjoy its soft feel and the ease with which you can deepen your stretch just by shifting your weight. The *Prerequisites* instruction refers you to a movement or exercise that you should be able to do *before* you undertake the selection on the page. Don't proceed unless you have mastered the forerunner.

Always feel free to use the *Power It Down* option as you begin your stability ball routine. When you're ready to increase the intensity, many of the instructions include ways to *Power It Up*.

Taking Size Into Consideration

The right size ball allows you to sit on it with your hips and knees bent at 90 degree angles. Unless your lower body is significantly longer than your upper body, you can choose a ball based on the following chart:

45 cm	Use if you are shorter than 5 feet tall
55 cm	Use if you are 5' to 5'7"
65 cm	Use if you are 5'8" to 6'2"
75 cm	Use if you are taller than 6'2"

When placing a stability ball *between* your legs, find one that opens your legs only about hip distance apart. If the ball is too large it may stress your hip and knee joints.

You may want to consider purchasing a *medicine ball* to use for exercises that call for a ball to be placed between your knees—its smaller size allows your hip joints to be in good alignment. They can also be purchased at different weights (3 pounds and up) to add intensity to your workout.

Some Safety Tips

- Use bare feet. This will give you better traction.
- Be on a padded surface. It's common to fall off the ball.
- Exercise away from objects or furniture you could bump into.
- If you have osteoporosis, or any recent injury, it would be advisable *not* to do any Ball exercises.

Pumping Up the Ball

- Beginners, keep the ball soft.
- Advanced exercisers, pump up the ball to be quite firm.

Taking Care of the Ball

- Keep the ball away from pointed or sharp objects.
- Don't wear jewelry or belts that could puncture the ball.
- Store the ball away from heat, including direct sunlight or lamps.

Get On the Ball

Be prepared to do a lot of squirming at first, as your body makes the necessary neuromuscular adjustments. True stabilization occurs when the ball does not move or roll as you perform an exercise. Don't be surprised if this does not come easily to you. Apply all the Pilates principles as you proceed—Navel to Spine, Kegels, lengthening, breathing. You will need to dig deep within yourself to create a heightened brain-to-muscle synergy.

With patience, persistence, and attention to the details and cueing instructions, you *will* succeed at conquering the ball.

Bridge

Level	Beginner
Purpose	Core stabilization (which is simultaneous strengthening of the abdominal and back muscles); strengthen the gluteals and the hamstrings
Prerequisite	Buttocks Squeeze, page 136

THE EXERCISES

Starting Position	Lie on your back with your lower legs on the ball, and your arms out to the sides, palms down.
Action	Exhale as you lift your pelvis up and form a straight line with your body. Inhale and return to the starting position.
Repetitions	Perform 8 times.

BODY CHECK

Head	Lengthen your neck so that your chin lowers slightly.
Shoulders	Keep your shoulders down by engaging your lats.
Arms/Hands	Your palms should be on the floor to help you stabilize.
Pelvis	Perform a Deep Abdominal Contraction. The challenge is to keep your hips level and not allow any movement of the ball.
Legs	Turn out from your hips by contracting the sides of your buttocks and the backs of your upper legs.

You Are Doing It Correctly if the ball does not move. Don't get discouraged; this may take some practice.

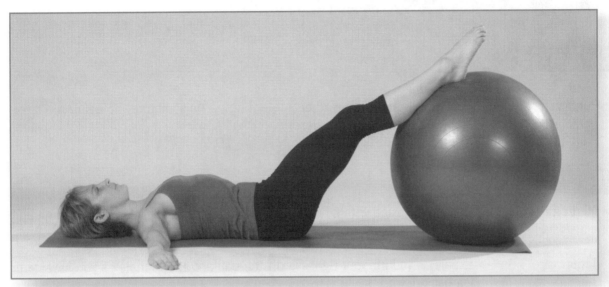

Starting Position: Lower legs on ball

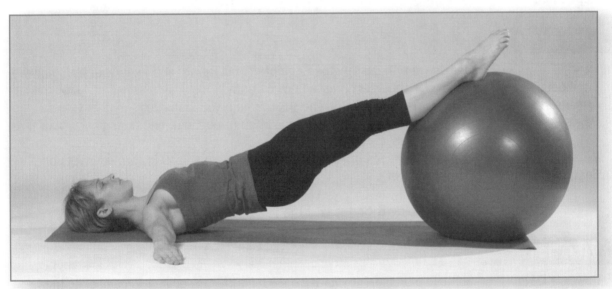

Action: Pelvis raised

Bridge with Leg Lift

Level	Intermediate
Purpose	Core stabilization; strengthen the entire leg musculature including the hamstrings, gluteals, and hip flexors
Prerequisites	Bridge, page 111; Leg Pull Front, page 162

THE EXERCISES

Starting Position	Lie on your back with both lower legs on the ball. Lift your hips up high and hold the position.
Action	Exhale as you lift your **right** leg off the ball and then inhale as you lower your leg back down.
Repetitions	Perform 5 successive repetitions with each leg.

BODY CHECK

Head	Imagine your head lengthening out of your spine, and keep your chin down.
Shoulders	Keep your shoulders pressed down gently.
Arms/Hands	Your palms should be on the floor to help you stabilize.
Pelvis	Maintain the bridge position, hips lifted throughout, and do not allow your hips to move in any direction.
Legs	Contract the sides of your buttocks and outer thighs to turn your legs out.
Feet	Point your feet.

You Are Doing It Correctly if the ball does not move.

VARIATIONS

Power It Down	Come to a bridge, lift your leg once, and then lower your torso back to the floor. Rest on the floor between each repetition.
Power It Up	Flex your foot as you lift your leg, and point your foot as you lower your leg.

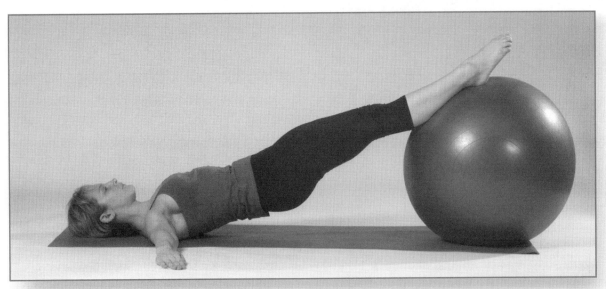

Starting Position: Pelvis raised

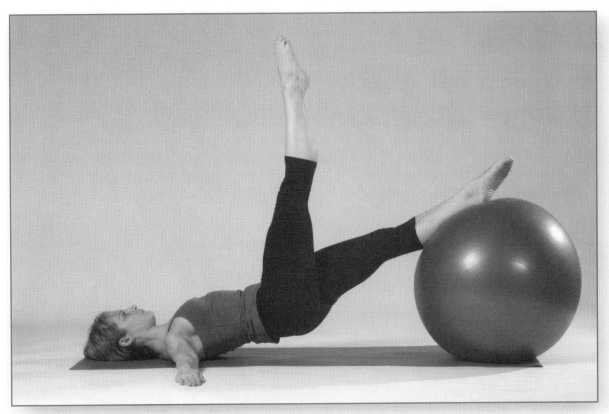

Action: Right leg lift

Teaser

Level	Intermediate
Purpose	Strengthen the abdominals
Prerequisite	Teaser I, page 140

THE EXERCISES

Starting Position	Lie on the floor with your lower legs on the ball and both arms extended overhead.
Action	Inhale and reach through your arms. Exhale, bring your arms over your chest and then lift your head and torso until you are balanced on your buttocks.
Repetitions	Perform 8 times.

BODY CHECK

Head	Keep your neck long.
Shoulders	Press your shoulders down.
Arms/Hands	Bring your arms up before you lift your head. Reach through your fingers and imagine your body lengthening through your arms and hands. This reaching should enable you to curl up higher and engage your abdominals more fully.
Pelvis	The impetus for this exercise emanates from your core; engage your abdominals and use your breathing. Avoid the temptation to swing your arms forcefully to propel yourself upward.

You Are Doing It Correctly if you move by contracting your abdominal muscles *and* not by flinging yourself up or using momentum.

VARIATIONS

Power It Down	Just lift your arms and your head off the floor.
Power It Up	Use wrist weights.

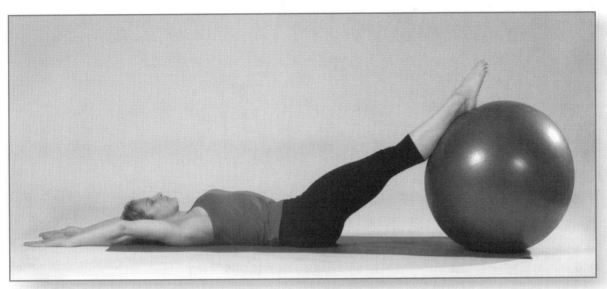

Starting Position: Lower legs on ball, arms overhead

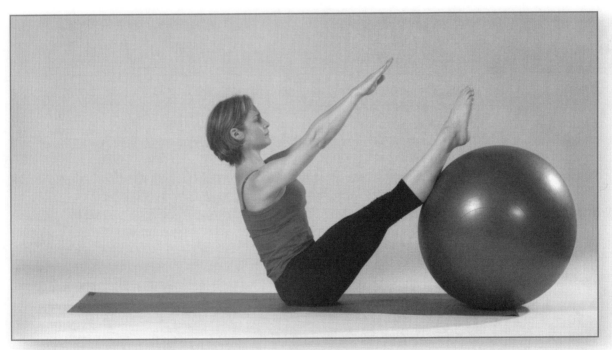

Action: Head and torso lift

Legs Lower and Lift

Level	Advanced
Purpose	Strengthen the abdominals; tone the inner thigh muscles
Prerequisite	Legs Lower and Lift, page 138

THE EXERCISES

Starting Position   Lie on your back holding a ball* between your lower legs. Raise your legs straight up in the air and place your hands behind your head. Lift your head off the floor and hold it there.

Action   Squeeze the ball with your inner thighs. Inhale and lower your legs. Keep squeezing the ball as you exhale and lift your legs to the starting position. (If you experience any pain, stop immediately).

Repetitions   Perform 5 times.

BODY CHECK

Head   Keep your head lifted throughout. If you need to lower your head, use the Power It Down suggestion.

Shoulders   Pay attention to keeping your shoulders pressed gently down.

Arms/Hands   Lightly touch the sides of your head or your ears with your fingers. Do not pull on your head with your hands.

Pelvis   Tighten your abdominals strongly to keep your back on the floor—do not allow your lower back to arch. Use your breathing.

Legs   Your legs should be in the Pilates Stance. Apply pressure on the ball by contracting your inner thigh muscles. When you bring your legs back up, be sure to return to the starting position and not beyond (not closer to your chest). Your legs should return to a position directly over your hip joints. Throughout the exercise, think of your legs reaching away from you, as if someone is tugging at your ankles.

You Are Doing It Correctly if your lower back does not move away from the floor as you lower your legs.

VARIATIONS

Power It Down   Keep your knees bent.

Power It Up   Lower your legs further down.

* Use a small stability ball or a medicine ball so that your legs are not spread too wide apart.

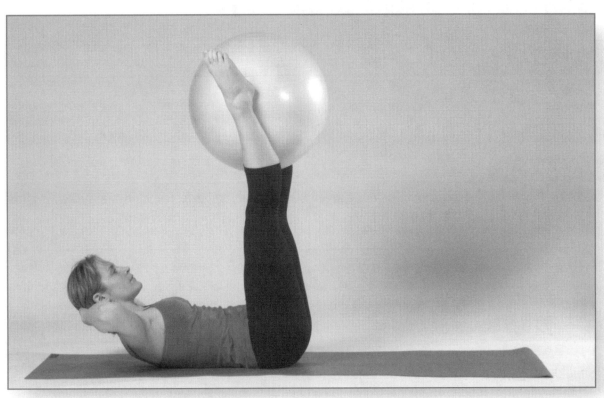

Starting Position: Legs straight up, head up

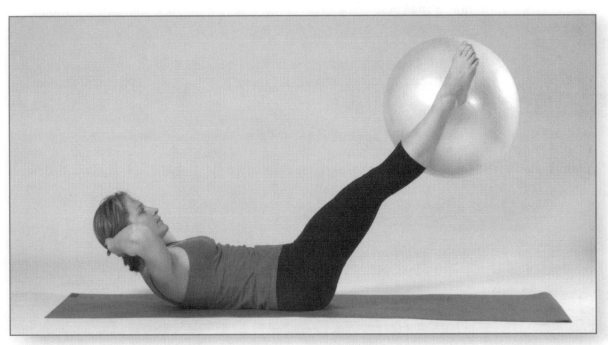

Action: Squeeze ball, legs lower

Corkscrew

AT A GLANCE

Level — Advanced
Purpose — Strengthen the abdominals
Prerequisite — Legs Lower and Lift, page 138

THE EXERCISES

Starting Position — Lean back on your forearms with your legs straight up in the air holding the ball*. (If you feel any pain in your back, stop immediately)

Action — Make a small, slow circle with your legs.

Repetitions — Circle 4 times in one direction, then circle 4 times in the other direction. Inhale as you begin the circle and exhale as you finish the circle.

BODY CHECK

Head — Keep your head and neck free of tension.
Shoulders — Don't sink down into your shoulders.
Arms/Hands — Press into your forearms and elbows to keep your chest lifted.
Pelvis — Your pelvis should not move. Keep your back in full contact with the floor during the circle using Deep Abdominal Contractions and your breathing.
Legs/Feet — Turn your legs out with your feet gently pointed.

You Are Doing It Correctly if your lower back remains in full contact with the floor throughout the exercise.

VARIATIONS

Power It Down — Remain in the Starting Position for a count of 10 while performing a Deep Abdominal Contraction.
Power It Up — Make a bigger circle, and pay close attention to maintaining pelvic stability.

* Use a smaller stability ball or a medicine ball.

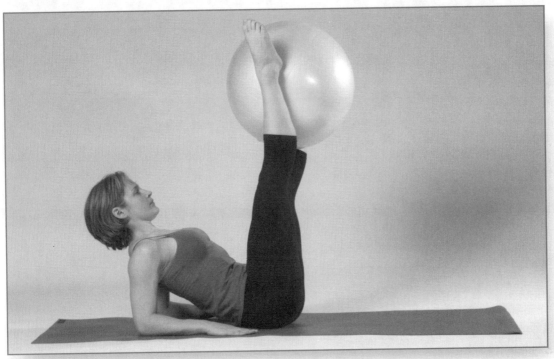

Starting Position: On forearms, legs straight up

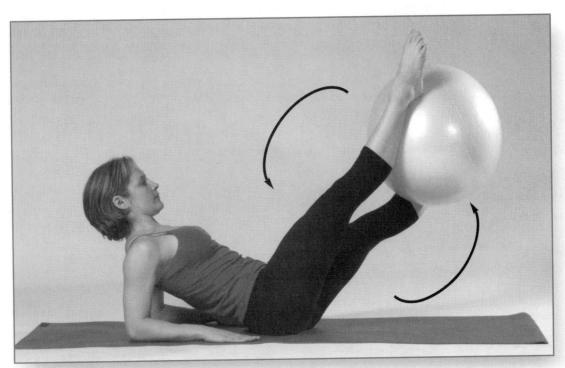

Action: Legs circle

Shoulder Stand with Leg Lift

AT A GLANCE

Level	Intermediate
Purpose	Core stabilization; strengthen gluteals, hamstrings, and hip flexors
Prerequisite	Bridge with Leg Lift, page 202

THE EXERCISES

Starting Position
Lie with your upper back on the ball, your hips raised, and your legs extended long on the floor. Keep your fingertips on the floor for support.

Action
Exhale as you lift your left leg, and inhale as you lower it and change legs.

Repetitions
Perform 8 sets (right and left counts as 1 set).

BODY CHECK

Head
Imagine your head lengthening out of your spine.

Shoulders
Keep them pressing down.

Arms/Hands
Place your fingertips (or hands) on the floor to help your stability.

Pelvis
The tendency will be for your hips to lower as your leg lifts. Generate power from your abdominals to maintain stability in your pelvis and prevent this from happening.

Legs
Turn your legs out from your hips by squeezing the sides of your buttocks. Lengthen out of your leg as you lift and lower.

Feet
Gently point your foot.

You Are Doing It Correctly if your hips stay in alignment *and* the ball does not move.

VARIATIONS

Power It Down
Remain in the Starting Position for a count of 10, with your abdominals strongly engaged. Rest, and then repeat.

Power It Up
Flex your foot as you lift your leg, and point your foot as you lower it.

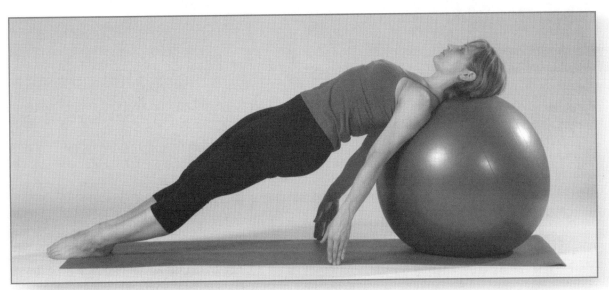

Starting Position: Upper back on ball, legs straight

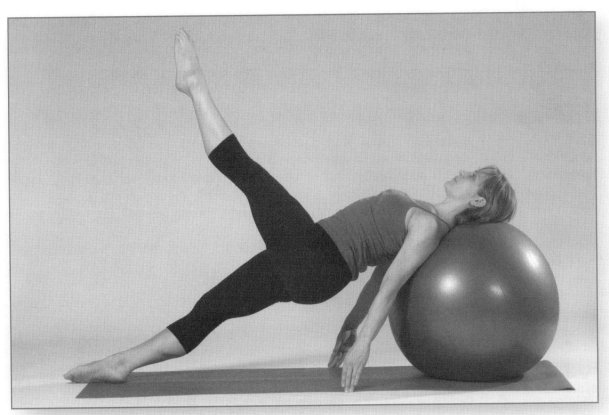

Action: Left leg lift

Side Leg Series

Level   Intermediate
Purpose   Tone the outer thighs
Prerequisites   Side Leg Series, page 164; Mermaid, page 168

THE EXERCISES

Starting Position   Begin on your knees with the ball to your **left** and your **left** forearm on the ball. Keep your torso lifted and lengthened out of your waist. Extend your **right** leg out to the side. Place your **right** hand on your waist.

Action   **1. Up and Down.** Exhale as you lift your **right** leg up and keep it parallel to the floor. Inhale as you lower your **right** leg.
2. Circle. Make small circles with your **right** leg, inhaling for two circles and exhaling for the next two.
3. Front and Back. Exhale as you flex your foot and bring your **right** leg to the front. Inhale, point your foot, and bring your leg to the back.

Repetitions   Perform 8 times with the right leg, then 8 times with the left.

BODY CHECK

Head   Imagine your head floating just above your spine.
Shoulders   Keep your shoulders down on your back.
Arms/Hands   Press into the ball with your **left** elbow and forearm to assist the lifting of your torso.
Pelvis   Strive to keep your hips as stable as possible; do not let them move up and down or forward and back.
Legs   Imagine your leg is lengthening as you lift, lower, move forward, back, and circle.

You Are Doing It Correctly if you keep your abdominals engaged *and* your upper body lifted.

VARIATIONS

Power It Up   Use ankle weights.

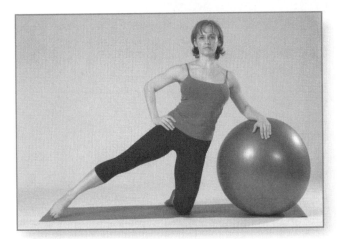

Starting Position: Left forearm on ball, right leg extended

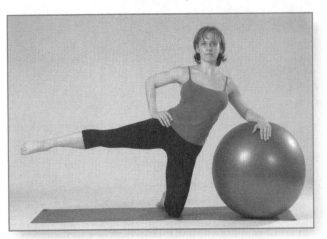

Action 1: Right leg lift

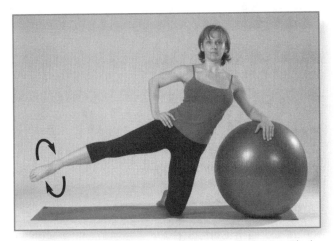

Action 2: Right leg circle

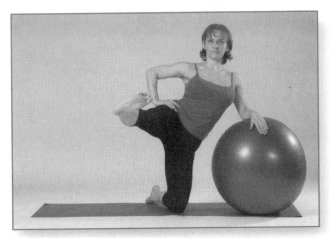

Action 3: Right leg extended forward

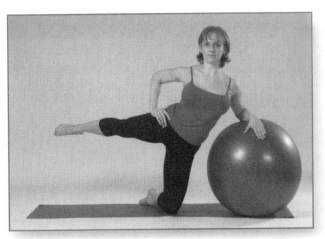

Action 3: Right leg extended backward

Walk the Hands

Level   Intermediate
Purpose   Core stabilization; strengthen the chest and arm muscles
Prerequisite   Push-Up Hold, page 170

THE EXERCISES

Starting Position   Begin with your stomach over the ball, your hands on the floor in front you, and your feet on the floor.

Action   "Walk" your hands forward on the floor so the ball slides down your legs, and then walk your hands back to the starting position.

Repetitions   Perform 5 sets (forward and back count as 1 set)

BODY CHECK

Head   Keep your head lifted so it stays aligned with your spine.
Shoulders   Your shoulders should be down.
Arms/Hands   Keep your hands shoulder width apart as you walk.
Pelvis   Strongly engage your abdominals.
Legs   Lengthen through your legs.

You Are Doing It Correctly if you feel you are one long line from your head to your toes *and* you walk forward to the point where your arms are supporting your body weight.

VARIATIONS

Power It Down   Walk forward and back once and then rest. Repeat until you have completed 5 sets.

Power It Up   Walk forward until the ball is supported by the tops of your ankles.

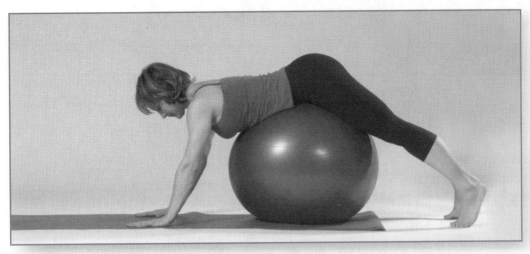

Starting Position: Stomach on ball, hands and toes on floor

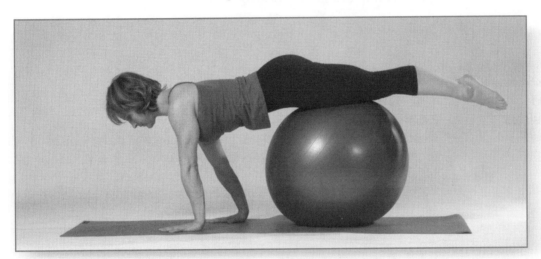

Action: Walk hands forward, legs off floor

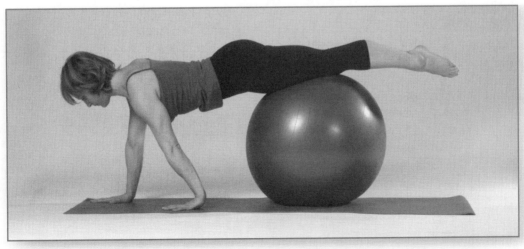

Action: Walk hands forward further

Push-Ups

Level	Intermediate
Purpose	Core stabilization; strengthen the chest and arm muscles
Prerequisites	Push-Ups, page 174; Walk the Hands, page 214

THE EXERCISES

Starting Position Place your upper legs on the ball and your hands* on the floor directly under your shoulders. Your feet should be off the floor.

Action Inhale, bend your elbows, and try to bring your chest close to the floor. Exhale and return to the starting position.

Repetitions Perform 8 times.

BODY CHECK

Head Your head should stay lifted and free of tension.

Shoulders Do not allow your shoulders to hunch up.

Arms/Hands Hand placement is very important in this exercise. Keep your hands directly under your shoulders, which may be closer together than you are accustomed to.

Pelvis Focus on maintaining core stabilization with your abdominals deeply contracted.

Legs Keep lengthening out through your legs.

You Are Doing It Correctly if you feel your arms supporting your weight *and* your body is in one straight line from head to toe.

VARIATIONS

Power It Down Perform fewer repetitions and only bend your elbows 2 to 3 inches.

Power It Up Place your toes or instep on the ball.

* Feel free to support your weight on your knuckles instead of your hands.

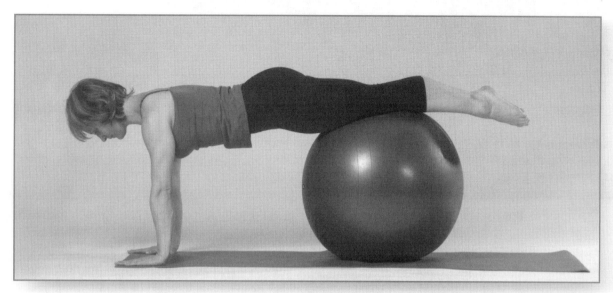

Starting Position: Upper legs on ball, hands on floor

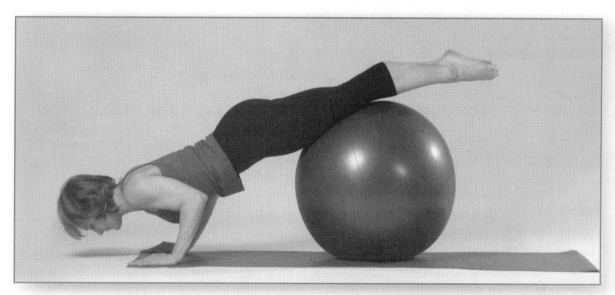

Action: Elbows bent, chest to floor

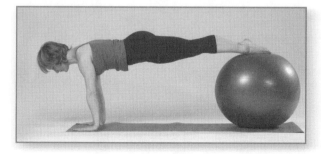

Power It Up: Insteps on ball

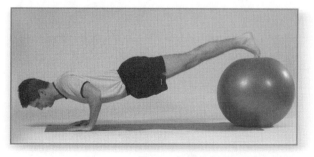

Power It Up 2: Toes on ball

Knee Tuck

Level	Intermediate
Purpose	Strengthen the lower fibers of the abdominals; isometrically strengthen the upper body
Prerequisite	Ball Push-Ups, page 216

THE EXERCISES

Starting Position	Place your hands on the floor in the Push-Up position, your lower legs on the ball, and your feet off the floor.
Action	Exhale as you bring your knees into your chest so your insteps are on the ball. Inhale, and return to the starting position.
Repetitions	Perform 8 times.

BODY CHECK

Head	Do not let your head droop; maintain proper alignment.
Shoulders	Press your shoulders down.
Arms/Hands	Your hands (or knuckles) should be directly under your shoulders.
Pelvis	Initiate the movement of the ball by using your abdominals, not by pushing on the floor.
Legs/Feet	Keep your legs and feet relaxed.

You Are Doing It Correctly if your upper body remains completely stationary as your legs move toward and away from you.

VARIATIONS

Power It Up	Perform 15 repetitions.

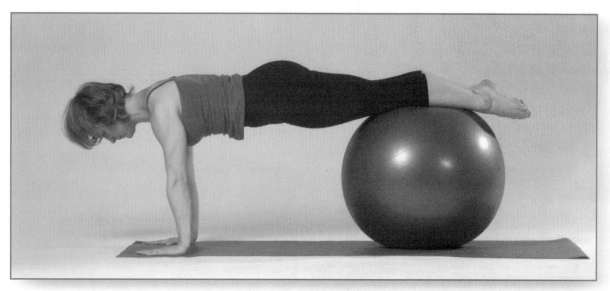

Starting Position: Lower legs on ball, hands on floor

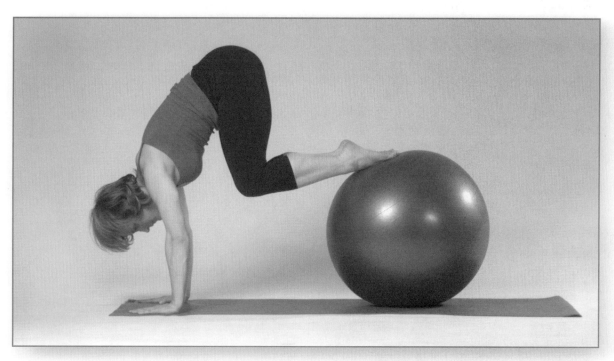

Action: Knees to chest, insteps on ball

Reverse Jackknife

Level	Advanced
Purpose	Strengthen the lower fibers of the abdominals; isometrically strengthen the upper body
Prerequisite	Knee Tuck, page 218

THE EXERCISES

Starting Position	Place your hands on the floor in the Push-Up position, your lower legs on the ball, and your feet off the floor.
Action	Exhale as you bring your legs in the direction of your chest and form an inverted V position. Inhale, and return to the starting position.
Repetitions	Perform 8 times.

BODY CHECK

Head	Do not let your head droop; maintain alignment.
Shoulders	Avoid letting your shoulders hunch up.
Arms/Hands	Keep your hands (or knuckles) placed directly under your shoulders.
Pelvis	Initiate the movement of the ball by using your abdominals, not by pushing on the floor.
Legs/Feet	Your legs should be in the Pilates Stance.

You Are Doing It Correctly if your upper body remains completely stationary as your legs move.

VARIATIONS

Power It Up	Perform the exercise with one leg lifted in the air. Alternate legs during the repetitions.

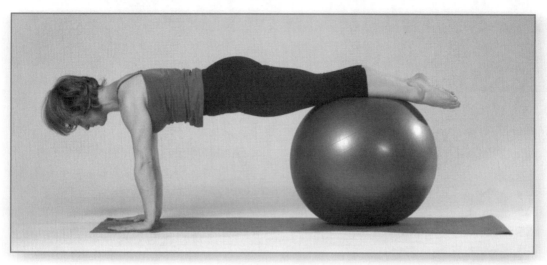

Starting Position: Lower legs on ball, hands on floor

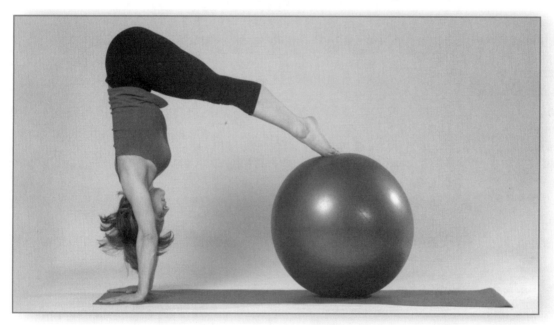

Action: Legs straight, inverted V position

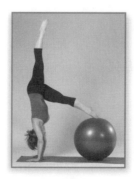

Power It Up: Left leg straight up

Leg Pull Back

Level	Advanced
Purpose	Strengthen the core, buttocks, and hamstrings; isometrically work the whole upper body
Prerequisite	Leg Pull Back, page 172

THE EXERCISES

Starting Position	Begin in the Push-Up position with your legs on the ball and your hands on the floor.
Action	Exhale as you lift your **left** leg up, and inhale as you lower it down.
Repetitions	Perform 5 times with the **right** leg and then 5 times with the **left**.

BODY CHECK

Head	Check that your head stays aligned with your spine and free of any tension.
Shoulders	Press your shoulders down.
Arms/Hands	Place your hands directly under your shoulders.
Pelvis	As your **left** leg lifts keep your **left** hip down, and vice versa. To do this strongly engage your abdominals throughout.
Legs/Feet	Lengthen through your legs.

You Are Doing It Correctly if the ball remains stationary.

VARIATIONS

Power It Up	Move the ball lower down on your leg.

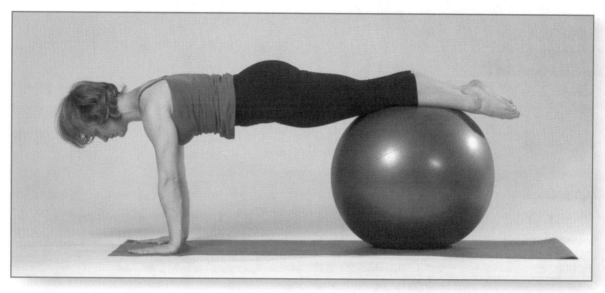

Starting Position: Push-Up position

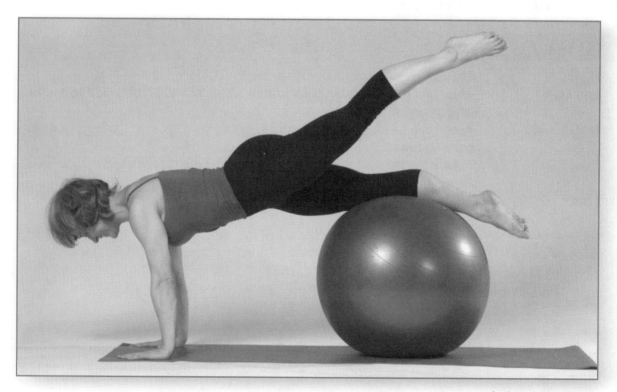

Action: Left leg lift

Reverse Hold

AT A GLANCE

Level	Advanced
Purpose	Strengthen the core, the back of your legs and isometrically work the whole upper body
Prerequisite	Leg Pull Front, page 162

THE EXERCISES

Starting Position	Sit on the floor with your legs on the ball. Lean back and put your hands on the floor with your fingers pointing forward*.
Action	Exhale as you lift your torso up until it is parallel to the floor. Inhale and return to the starting position.
Repetitions	Hold for a slow count of 10. Lower. Then repeat.

BODY CHECK

Head	Think of your head as a natural extension of your spine.
Shoulders	Press into your hands to keep your shoulders down. Do not allow your shoulders to hunch up.
Arms/Hands	Keep your hands positioned directly under your shoulders with your fingers pointing toward your body.
Pelvis	Initiate the movement with a Deep Abdominal Contraction and lift your pelvis as one unit to form a straight line from your head to your toes.
Legs	Feel that your legs are lengthening away from you.

You Are Doing It Correctly if you feel the work in your abdominals and not only in your arms.

* Or you can support yourself on your knuckles.

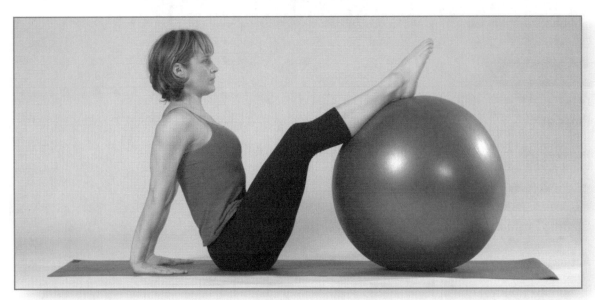

Starting Position: Legs on ball, fingers pointing forward

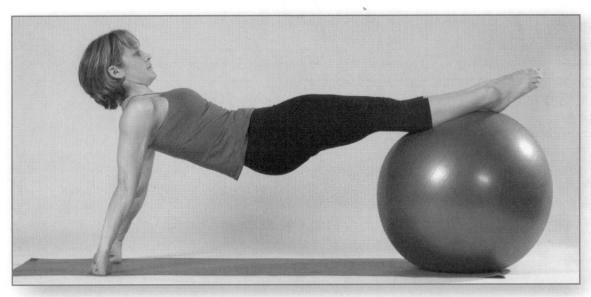

Action: Torso lift on knuckles

Opposite Arm and Leg Lift

AT A GLANCE

Level	Beginner
Purpose	Strengthen your upper, middle, and lower back; strengthen your hamstrings and buttocks muscles
Prerequisite	Opposite Arm and Leg Lift, page 184

THE EXERCISES

Starting Position	Lay with your torso over the ball, and your hands and feet on the floor.
Action	Exhale as you simultaneously lift and lengthen your **right** arm and **left** leg. (Be sure it's the *opposite* arm and leg). Then switch sides.
Repetitions	Perform 8 sets (right and left count as 1 set).

BODY CHECK

Head	Keep your head lifted and steady. Do not allow your head to bob up and down.
Shoulders	Press your shoulders down on your back.
Arms/Hands	Lengthen out of your arm as you lift and as you lower.
Pelvis	Engage your abdominals to stabilize your pelvis.
Legs	Lengthen out of your leg as you lift and as you lower.

You Are Doing It Correctly if the ball does not move.

VARIATIONS

Power It Up	Perform 12 sets. You can also use ankle and wrist weights.

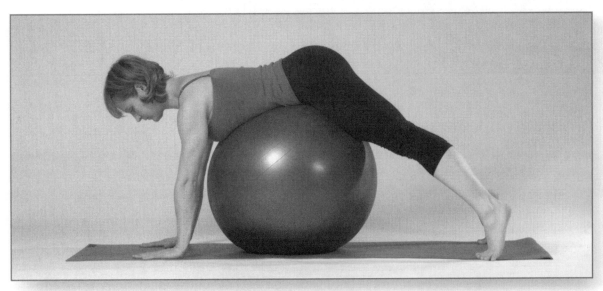

Starting Position: Torso on ball

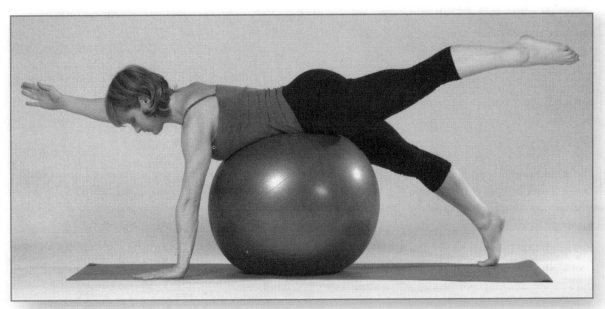

Action: Right arm and left leg lift

Swan

Level	Advanced
Purpose	Strengthen the back
Prerequisites	Swan, page 180; Flight, page 182

THE EXERCISES

Starting Position Place the ball under your hips. Rest your feet on the floor, keep your legs straight and your arms outstretched in front of you.

Action Inhale as you lift up, reach your arms forward and then up, and allow your back to arch. Exhale, and return to the starting position.

Repetitions Perform 5 times.

BODY CHECK

Head Allow your head to move naturally as an extension of your spine. Do not throw your head back.

Shoulders Engage your lats to keep your shoulders down.

Arms/Hands Reach through your fingers.

Pelvis Feel the energy for this exercise centered in your core.

Legs Keep your legs straight.

You Are Doing It Correctly if you feel the lengthening as you slowly lift and lower *and* you are not hurling your body upwards with momentum.

VARIATIONS

Power It Down Keep your arms by your sides and just lift your upper body.

Power It Up Hold a Magic Ring with your arms outstretched.

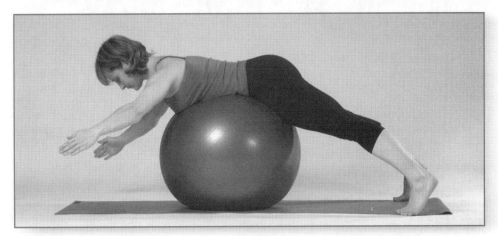

Starting Position: Hips on ball, legs straight

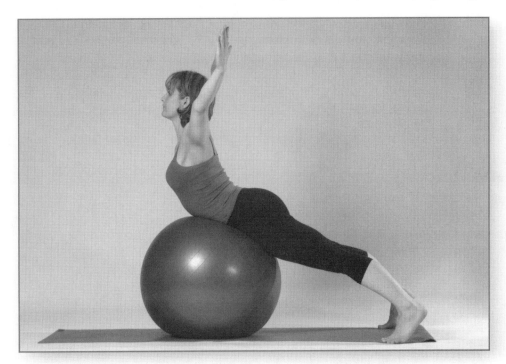

Action: Torso lift, arms up

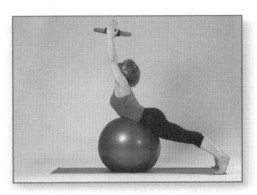

Power It Up: Torso lift with Magic Ring

Ball Stretches: Back Arch

Level	All levels (However, if you have a back or neck problem, avoid this stretch).
Purpose	Stretch the whole front of the body, including the abdominals and chest; improve the flexibility of the spine in extension
Prerequisite	Head Drop Back, page 72

THE EXERCISES

Starting Position Sit on the ball.

Action Push out with your feet so that your legs straighten as you reach your arms overhead. You will be performing a back bend over the ball. Let your head relax and your chest lift.

Repetitions Hold for a count of 5. Keep breathing. With each exhale increase the stretch. Return to the starting position for a moment, and then repeat the stretch.

BODY CHECK

This should feel great. If there's any pain—stop immediately.

Think of reaching through your fingers to elongate your spine.

Take your eyes along for the stretch—look up and back to see if this increases your ability to arch.

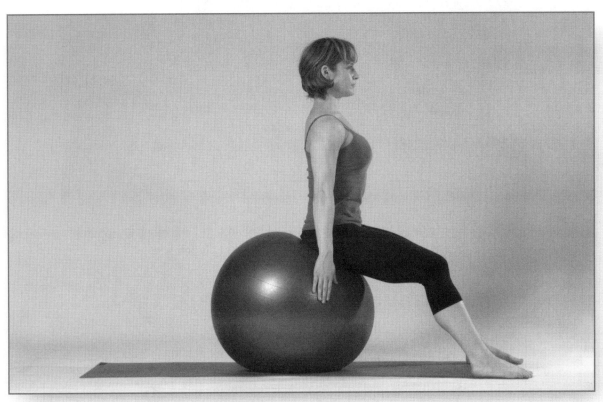

Starting Position: Seated on ball

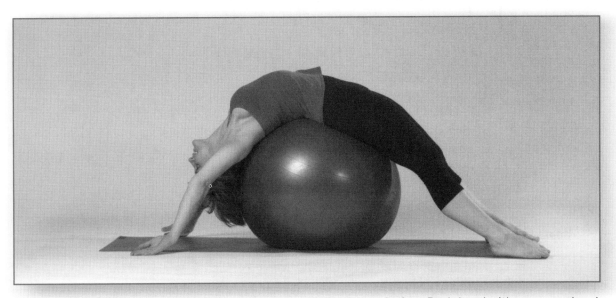

Action: Back bend with arms overhead

Ball Stretches: Twist

Level	All levels
Purpose	Improve the ability of the spine to perform rotation
Prerequisites	Seated Twist, page 154; Rotation, page 66

THE EXERCISES

Starting Position Sit on the ball and hold a Magic Ring* out in front of you.

Action Turn your upper body to the **right** and hold the position. Keep your hips facing forward. Then twist to the **left** and hold the stretch.

Repetitions Keep breathing as you hold the stretch for a slow count of 5 in each direction. Use each exhalation as an opportunity to increase the stretch.

BODY CHECK

Keep your shoulders down.
Avoid changing the distance between your arms (this is what happens most often). The twist should come from your spine and not from your arms.
Move your head and eyes in the same direction you are turning.
Pay attention to your hips; they stay facing forward.

* If you do not have a Magic Ring, bring both arms out to your sides.

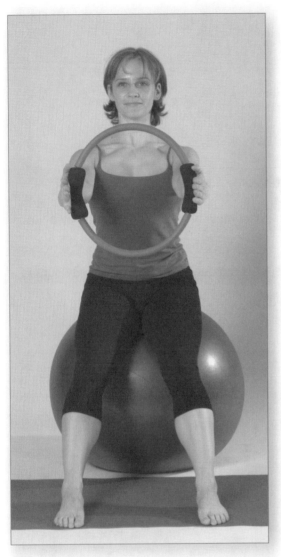

Starting Position: Sitting on ball holding
Magic Ring in front

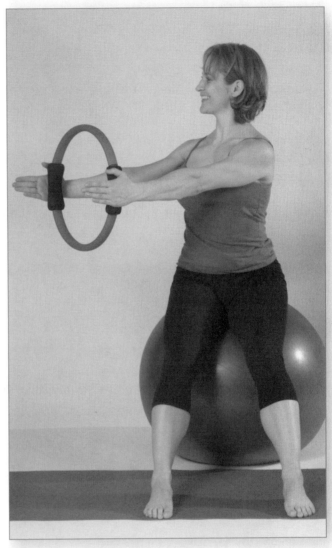

Action: Hips facing forward, torso twist right

Ball Stretches: Side Stretch

Level	All levels
Purpose	Stretch the lats, waistline, and side of the hips
Prerequisite	Lifting Up While Sitting, page 56

THE EXERCISES

Starting Position	Sit on the ball with your feet apart holding a Magic Ring* overhead.
Action	Bend your whole torso to the **left** as you move the ball to the **right** with your pelvis.
Repetitions	Hold for a slow count of 10. Pause for a moment and then repeat. Be sure to perform the stretch on both sides.

BODY CHECK

Keep reaching through your fingers.

Feel a sense of lengthening out of your waist.

Remember to focus on your breathing; with each exhalation take the stretch to a new point of gentle tension.

* If you do not have a Magic Ring, reach both arms overhead.

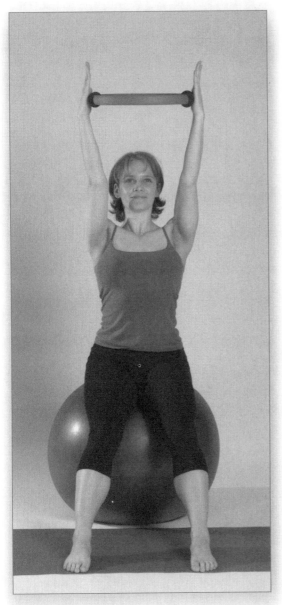

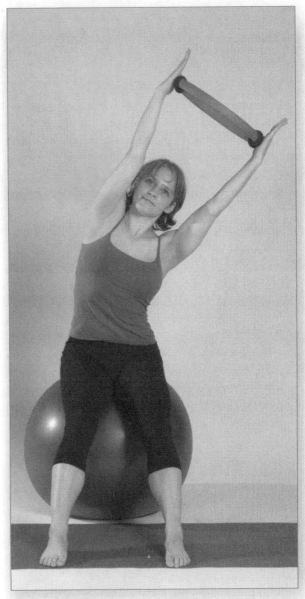

Starting Position: Sitting on ball holding
Magic Ring overhead

Action: Torso bend left

Ball Stretches: Shoulder Stretch

AT A GLANCE

Level	All levels
Purpose	Stretch the shoulders and upper back
Prerequisite	Lifting Up While Sitting, page 56

THE EXERCISES

Starting Position   Sit on the ball and hold a Magic Ring* over your head.

Action   Tuck your pelvis under as you bring your arms down in front of you and push them away slightly. Bring your arms back up overhead as you tilt your pelvis in the other direction and return to the starting position.

Repetitions   Perform slowly 5 times.

BODY CHECK

Perform a pelvic tilt, forward and back, to increase the stretch in each position.
Reach through your arms but keep your shoulders down.
As you hold the stretch, continue to breathe in and out. Each time you exhale gently increase your stretch.

* Or interlace your fingers and press your palms toward the ceiling.

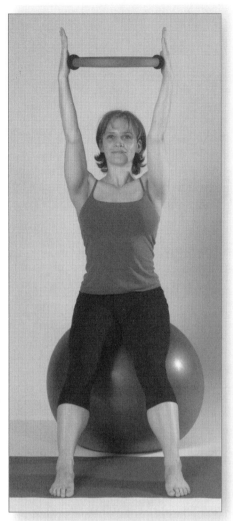

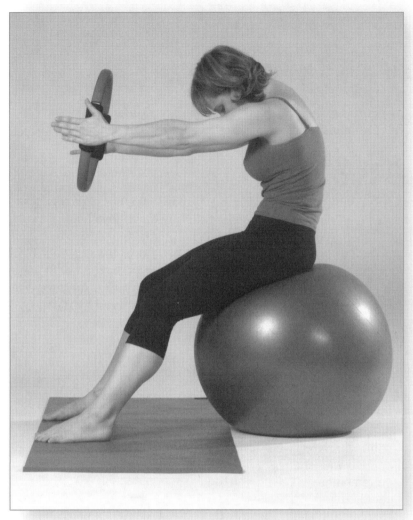

Starting Position: Sitting on ball, holding Magic Ring overhead

Action: Arms down in front, pelvis tucked under

Ball Stretches: Hamstring Stretch

AT A GLANCE

Level	All levels
Purpose	Stretch the hamstrings
Prerequisite	Hamstring Flexibility, page 84

THE EXERCISES

Starting Position   Place your **left** hand on a sturdy support and your **right** leg on the ball. Bring your **right** arm straight overhead.

Action   Exhale and bend over towards your **right** leg with a straight back. Allow your **right** arm to move as one unit with your spine and keep reaching out through your **right** hand. Tilt your pelvis away *slightly* so that your lower back arches a little. Hold for a slow count of 10. Keep breathing, and with each exhale gently increase the stretch.

Repetitions   Hold for a slow count of 10.

BODY CHECK

Your leg and arm should stay as straight and extended as possible.
Imagine energy projecting outward from your fingertips.
Keep your shoulders relaxed.
Remember to breathe.

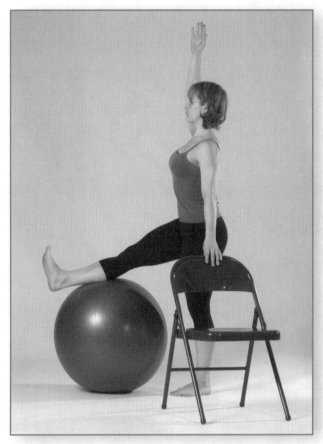 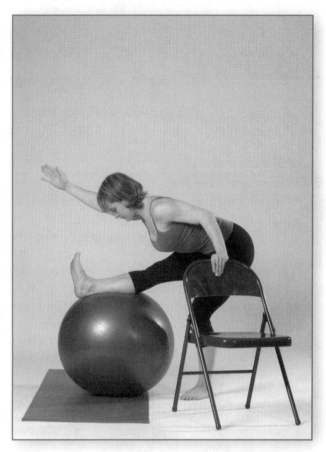

Starting Position: Right leg on ball, right arm overhead

Action: Bend down, right arm straight

Ball Stretches: Inner Thigh Stretch

AT A GLANCE

Level	All levels
Purpose	Stretch the inner thighs
Prerequisite	Inner Thigh flexibility, Page 86

THE EXERCISES

Starting Position   Stand so you can hold onto a stable support with the ball beside your **right** leg. Place your **right** heel on top of the ball. Keep both legs turned out from your hips so your feet also turn out slightly.

Action   Bend your **left** knee to increase the stretch of your **right** inner thigh. Hold for a slow count of 10, and with each breath try to increase the range of motion to get a deeper stretch.

Repetitions   Hold for a count of 10 with each leg.

BODY CHECK

Make sure your standing leg is turned out.
Scan your body for any tension, especially in the neck and shoulders.
Keep breathing.

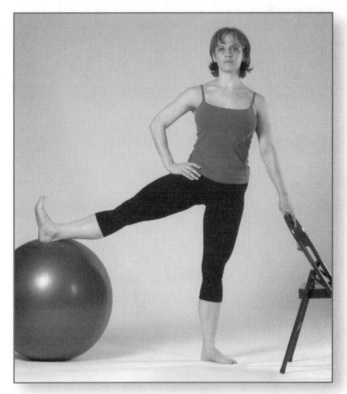

Starting Position: Right heel on ball

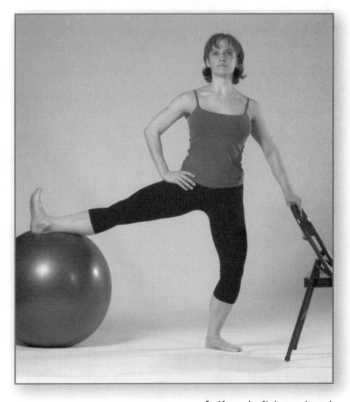

Action: Left knee bend

Ball Stretches: Hip Flexor Stretch

AT A GLANCE

Level	All levels
Purpose	Stretch the front of the leg and groin area
Prerequisite	Hip Flexor Flexibility, page 88

THE EXERCISES

Starting Position Hold onto a wall or sturdy support. With the ball behind you place your **right** instep on the ball.

Action Push the ball away from you with your **right** leg and bend both knees to sink down into your hips. Feel the stretch along the front of your **right** thigh and groin area. Hold for a slow count of 10. Keep breathing and with each exhale gently increase the stretch.

Repetitions Perform twice with each leg.

BODY CHECK

Your shoulders remain down.
Keep your neck tension free.

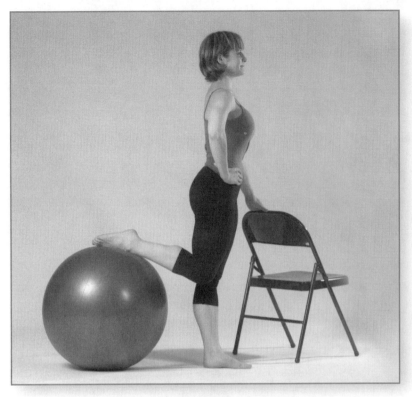

Starting Position: Right instep on ball

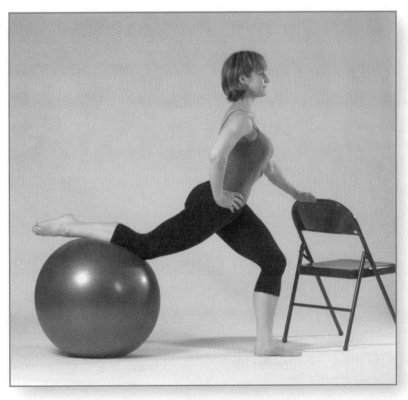

Action: Left knee bent, right leg back

Chapter 10

The Pilates Perfect Workouts

Beginner

Your future development as a Pilates student begins with this program. Maximize its benefits by paying careful attention to all instructions and moving slowly through the series. This will greatly reduce your risk of injury and muscle soreness while providing you the opportunity to cultivate your skills.

Try to do the program three times a week with at least one day of rest in between. Start with the lowest number of repetitions *(Min Reps)* listed, and progressively increase to the higher number *(Max Reps)*. Feel free to rest and stretch your muscles as often as you need to. Refer back to Chapter 7: *The Release Movements*, for more ideas that can be integrated into your program.

If you are a newcomer to the Pilates method you may benefit by continuing with this program for one to three months before moving on.

Although Ball exercises are included, you will still feel the effects of a complete workout even if you choose not to purchase this piece of equipment.

Mat Exercises	Page	Min Reps	Max Reps
Breathing to 100	120	100	100
Roll Up	122	6	8
Bridge	111	1	1
Single Knee Stretch	124	6	10
Pilates First*(Power It Down)	132	6	10
Straight Leg Stretch	128	6	10
Buttocks Squeeze	136	6	10
Inner Thigh Curl*(Power It Down)	134	6	10
Leg Circles	144	4	8

Teaser I*(Power It Down)	140	4	8
Spine Stretch	152	2	4
Reverse Hold*(Power It Down)	160	2	4
Side Leg Series	164	4	8
Push-Up Hold	170	2	4
4 Points	176	4	8
4 Points Leg Series	178	4	8
Swan	180	1	1
Prayer Stretch	112	1	1
Flight	182	4	8
Opposite Arm and Leg Lift	184	4	10
Cat Stretch	194	3	3
Full Body Stretch	104	1	1

Ball Exercises	Page	Min Reps	Max Reps
Bridge	200	4	8
Teaser * (Power It Down)	204	4	8
Walk the Hands	214	4	8
Opposite Arm and Leg Lift	226	4	8

Ball Stretches	Page	Min Reps	Max Reps
Back Arch	230	1	1
Twist	232	1	1
Side Stretch	234	1	1
Shoulder Stretch	236	1	1
Hamstring Stretch	238	1	1
Inner Thigh Stretch	240	1	1

* Be sure to begin with the Power it Down version

Intermediate

When you are able to perform the exercises in the Beginner program with ease and assurance, it's time to add to your repertoire and intensity. You'll enjoy the novelty of new movements and notice that you are being challenged to a higher level of fitness and body awareness.

Be sure to stretch after each exercise you perform lying on your stomach. You may incorporate as many rest intervals as you feel you need without compromising the benefits of any part of the workout.

There may not always be an increase in the number of repetitions as you advance through the workout levels. The added intesity is created by the combination and commulative effect of the exercises.

The Mat exercises listed below stand by themselves as a full body program; the stability ball segments are supplemental. Use the Power It Down options as needed, and before you move on to the Advanced program, be sure to try the Power It Up suggestions.

Mat Exercises	Page	Min Reps	Max Reps
Breathing to 100	120	100	100
Roll Up	122	8	10
Single Knee Stretch	124	8	10
Double Leg Extension	126	4	8
Side to Side Rocking	106	1	1
Straight Leg Stretch	128	8	10
90/90	130	4	8
Leg Circles	144	4	8
Pilates First	132	4	8
Inner Thigh Curl	134	4	8
Buttocks Squeeze	136	20	20
Teaser I	140	4	8
Spine Stretch	152	4	4
Seated Twist	154	4	4
Rolling Like A Ball	156	4	6
Roll Down	158	2	6

Reverse Hold	160	4	8
Side Leg Series	164	8	12
Side Stretch	166	1	1
4 Points Leg Series	178	8	12
Swan	180	1	1
Flight	182	8	1
Prayer Stretch	112	1	1
Double Leg Lift	188	6	10
Hip Shake	113	4	4
Swimming	186	8	12
Quad Stretch	190	1	1
Cat Stretch	194	3	3
Full Body Stretch	104	1	1

Ball Exercises	Page	Min Reps	Max Reps
Bridge with Leg Lift	202	4	8
Teaser	204	4	8
Shoulder Stand with Leg Lift	210	4	8
Push-Ups	216	4	8
Knee Tuck	218	4	8
Opposite Arm and Leg Lift	226	4	8
Swan*(Power It Down)	228	3	5

Ball Stretches	Page	Min Reps	Max Reps
Back Arch	230	2	2
Twist	232	2	2
Side Stretch	234	2	2
Shoulder Stretch	236	2	2
Hamstring Stretch	238	2	2
Inner Thigh Stretch	240	2	2
Hip Flexor Stretch	242	2	2

Advanced

If you are preparing to begin the Advanced program, you should be proud of yourself for having achieved a high degree of grace and athletic ability.

If you regularly engage in sports, this program will augment your training regimen and give you exceptional core stability that may translate into better performance. Your workout intensity will not be dimnished if you rest between exercises (review Chapter 7).

You are on your way to complete mastery of the most difficult Pilates exercises and will soon feel the power that emanates from a body and mind working in harmony.

Mat Exercises	Page	Min Reps	Max Reps
Roll Up	122	10	12
Single Knee Stretch	124	10	12
Double Leg Extension	126	8	10
Straight Leg Stretch	128	10	12
90/90	130	8	10
Side to Side Rocking	106	1	1
Pilates First	132	8	10
Inner Thigh Curl	134	8	10
Buttocks Squeeze	136	20	20
Legs Lower and Lift	138	4	8
Leg Circles	144	4	8
Teaser II	142	4	6
Crisscross	146	4	8
Scissors	148	4	8
Spine Stretch	152	4	4
Seated Twist	154	4	4
Rolling Like A Ball	156	4	6
Roll Down	158	4	6
Leg Pull Front	162	4	8
Side Leg Series	164	8	12
Mermaid	168	1	1

4 Points Leg Series	178	8	12
Swan	180	1	1
Flight	182	8	12
Prayer Stretch	112	1	1
Double Leg Lift	188	8	12
Hip Shake	113	4	4
Swimming	186	8	12
Quad Stretch	190	1	1
Rocking	192	2	4
Cat Stretch	194	3	3
Full Body Stretch	104	1	1

Ball Exercises	Page	Min Reps	Max Reps
Legs Lower and Lift	206	4	8
Corkscrew	208	4	8
Side Leg Series	212	8	12
Reverse Jackknife	220	4	8
Leg Pull Back	222	4	8
Reverse Hold	224	1	2
Opposite Arm and Leg Lift	226	8	12
Swan	228	4	6

Ball Stretches	Page	Min Reps	Max Reps
Back Arch	230	2	2
Twist	232	2	2
Side Stretch	234	2	2
Shoulder Stretch	236	2	2
Hamstring Stretch	238	2	2
Inner Thigh Stretch	240	2	2
Hip Flexor Stretch	242	2	2

Chapter 11

Strategies for Improving

*T*he beauty of Pilates is that it is an ongoing quest. You can always enhance the intensity, execution and technique to meet your new level of fitness. Developing your inner strength, both physical and mental, can be a lifetime's work.

If you feel you have hit a plateau and are not seeing the improvements you crave, try these tips.

- First of all, don't try to "barrel through" the exercises. Most likely you will be using momentum, instead of your muscles. Go slower, not faster.

- Instead of doing more, do less—decrease the range of motion. Don't raise your head so far off the floor, or lift your legs so high. Do fewer repetitions, and rest more. Take a look at the *Power It Down* option for each exercise. Your goal is quality, not quantity.

- Go inward. Put all your effort into making the contractions in your belly and pelvic floor stronger. It is the internal effort, that which is invisible, that will change you most.

- Pay attention to the breathing instructions. Use your breath as a force to mobilize your body. You will immediately feel a heightened awareness and ability to engage your abdominals more powerfully.

- Spend more time with Chapter 6: *The Secrets to Good Pilates Technique*. Instead of just doing the repetitions suggested, do more, perhaps double the amount. The key to this chapter is going very slowly and using small, almost imperceptible movements as you begin the sequences. It takes time to readjust our normal inclination to always work "hard." An instruction to do a movement with the *least* amount of effort possible seems counterintuitive, but it is the right path to the destination you seek.

- Go back to Chapter 4: *Learning the Basics*. See if you can uncover new meaning in the directions that will help you make stronger connections between thought and action.

You may want to try some local Pilates classes. Be selective if you have an array to choose from. Here is what to look for:

- There should be a running commentary throughout the class by the instructor; he or she should be talking almost continuously.

- Are you getting frequent reminders to reinforce proper technique? Is your attention repeatedly being directed to your breathing, your abdominals, and your alignment? Some of the verbal cues you might hear are: "keep your shoulders relaxed," "bring your navel to your spine," "lengthen through your arms," "keep your neck free of tension," and "stay focused on your breathing."

- "Hands-on" corrections by the teacher are vital. While not every student will be touched by the instructor in class, you must get these tactile cues from time to time to ensure you are correctly engaging your muscles and properly aligning your body.

Finally, I urge you to find out more about Feldenkrais. If ever there were a fountain of youth, this would certainly be it. For some people, the movements in Chapter 6 will not achieve the desired improvements. Each of us is built differently, with body parts that have a unique way of moving, or of not being able to move. The short Feldenkrais mini-processes in this book may not be targeted enough to meet your specific needs.

There are two paths you can take:

- Awareness Through Movement® classes are taught to groups of people at one time. They are led by a single teacher who verbally instructs the class through a series of pleasurable, playful, and revealing movements. They will be similar to what you see in Chapter 6, but much longer. This gives your body additional options to choose from and more time to undo restrictive patterns. Try your local YMCA, community center, or health club to experience one of these classes.

- Functional Integration® is the "hands on" component of the method. This is a one-on-one approach that will be targeted specifically to your body and your needs. You will be asked to sit or lie, fully clothed, while gentle pressure is applied by a Feldenkrais practitioner. After about an hour you will stand up and see if you can recognize and appreciate what your body has just learned. Perhaps you will hold yourself in a new way, or your ability to move will have dramatically improved; there may be a new springiness in your joints; you may feel your feet growing roots into the ground; a limitation you previously had may be gone—the possibilities are endless. The only drawback is that these individual sessions can be quite pricey. You can expect to pay $80 or more for a Feldenkrais lesson. It takes nearly four years of training and study to become a certified Feldenkrais practitioner.

- Contact the Feldenkrais Guild at the telephone number or website listed in the Addendum for further information. They can direct you to nearby group classes and individual practitioners.

Be grateful to your body for taking you this far in life. Pilates will bring forth the power that still lies within you.

List of Exercises

chapter 8 — The Mat Exercises

Breathing to 100
Roll Up
Single Knee Stretch
Double Leg Extension
Straight Leg Stretch
90/90
Pilates First
Inner Thigh Curl
Buttocks Squeeze
Legs Lower and Lift
Teaser I
Teaser II
Leg Circles
Crisscross
Scissors
Rollover
Spine Stretch
Seated Twist
Rolling Like A Ball
Roll Down
Reverse Hold
Leg Pull Front
Side Leg Series
Side Stretch
Mermaid
Push-Up Hold
Leg Pull Back
Push-Ups
4 Points
4 Points Leg Series
Swan
Flight
Opposite Arm and Leg Lift
Swimming
Double Leg Lift
Quad Stretch
Rocking
Cat Stretch

chapter 9 — The Ball Exercises

Bridge
Bridge with Leg Lift
Teaser
Legs Lower and Lift
Corkscrew
Shoulder Stand with Leg Lift
Side Leg Series
Walk the Hands
Push-Ups
Knee Tuck
Reverse Jackknife
Leg Pull Back
Reverse Hold
Opposite Arm and Leg Lift
Swan

The Ball Stretches

Back Arch
Twist
Side Stretch
Shoulder Stretch
Hamstring Stretch
Inner Thigh Stretch
Hip Flexor Stretch

Glossary

Core. The muscles encircling your midsection: front, side, and back.

Deep Abdominal Contraction. Exhale as you pull your navel straight back toward your spine and perform a Kegel. Do not tuck your pelvis under.

Engage the lats. Contract the muscles below your shoulder blades in a downward direction.

Exhale. Expel air fully through your mouth. Think of completely deflating your lungs.

Expand your rib cage or expand your ribs like a ball. Your ribs are in the front, side and all around the back of your body. When you breathe, fill your ribs with air as if you were inflating a big ball.

Flex the foot. Bring your foot toward your shin. Don't curl your toes. Reach through your heel bone.

Head in neutral alignment. Your chin should not be reaching forward. Feel your head as a natural extension of your spine. Pay close attention to alignment in the pictures.

Hip Flexors. The collective term for the group of muscles along the front of your hip and thigh.

Gluteals. Your buttocks muscles.

Inhale. Take a deep breath through your nose and expand your rib cage. Think of the breath coming from your lungs.

Instep. The top surface of the arch of your foot, between your ankle and your toes.

Isometric. A type of muscular contraction where there is no visible movement, yet you feel tension building. Example: pressing your hands strongly together and holding it.

Isotonic. Type of muscular contraction in which the muscle shortens and lengthens. Example: bending and straightening at the elbow which uses the biceps muscles.

Kegel. Contract the muscles that stop the flow of urine. You should be "pulling up" the pelvic floor.

Lats. The common term for the *latissimus dorsi*, a large muscle of your back, situated from the bottom of your shoulder blades all the way to the top of your buttocks.

Lengthen out of the arms/fingers. Feel as though someone has hold of your wrists and is trying to pull your arms out of your shoulder sockets.

Lengthen out of the legs. Feel as though someone has hold of your ankles and is trying to pull your legs out of your hip sockets.

Lengthen out of the waist. Increase the distance between your hip bones and your bottom rib; get taller; create space between the vertebrae.

Navel to spine. Pull your belly button straight in. Deeply contract your abdominals without any movement of your pelvis.

Pelvic tilt or tuck. When your lower back presses down into the floor your hips move. For abdominal strengthening, avoid this.

Pilates stance. Turn your legs out from your hips. Squeezing the sides of your buttocks and upper legs.

Point the foot. Move your foot away from your shin. Don't curl your toes under. Feel a stretch at the top arch of your foot, or instep.

Reach through the arms/hands. Feel as though someone has hold of your wrists and is trying to pull your arms out of your shoulder sockets.

Reach through the legs. Feel as though someone has hold of your ankles and is trying to pull your legs out of your hip sockets.

Shoulders down and relaxed. Do a mild contraction of the lats which brings your shoulder blades down.

Stabilize the pelvis. Do not allow your pelvis to move in any direction. Perform a Deep Abdominal Contraction by bringing your navel to your spine while performing a Kegel. Your upper back does not move at all.

Stabilize the spine. Feel like your torso is anchored to the floor. Use your lats to move your shoulder blades downward. Your lower back does not move at all.

Turn out from the hips. Squeeze the sides of your buttocks and upper thighs. Do not initiate from the feet.

Resources

Pilates Products & Certifications
The Xercize Corporation
800-IMX-1336
www.Xercize.com

Feldenkrais® Information
Feldenkrais Guild of North America
800-775-2118
503-221-6612
FAX 503-221-6616
www.feldenkrais.com

Exercise Equipment
GetFitNow.com
800-906-1234
www.getfitnow.com

Perform Better Catalogue
www.performbetter.com
800-556-7464

Power Systems Catalogue
800-321-6975
www.power-systems.com

About the Author

Dianne Daniels, MA, has a masters degree in exercise physiology from Columbia University. A former health educator with the New York City Department for Aging, she has developed exercise programs for individuals of all ages. A Feldenkrais® practitioner, Pilates instructor, Yoga teacher, and personal trainer, Ms. Daniels has taught academic and practical courses for fitness professionals since 1992.

Also by the Author:

Exercises for Osteoporosis, Revised Edition (Hatherleigh Press, 2004)

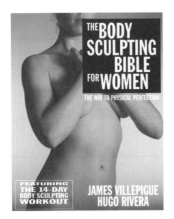
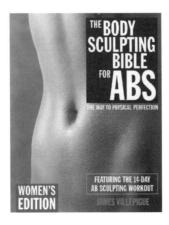
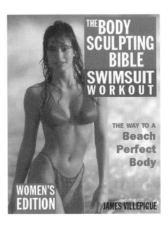

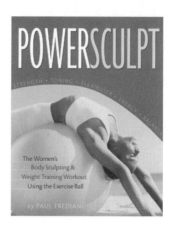
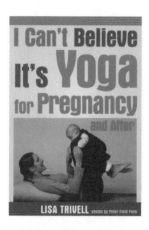
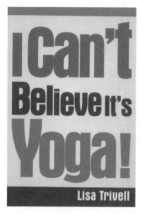
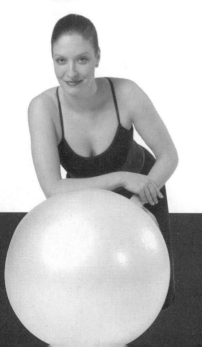

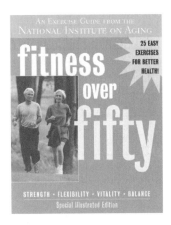
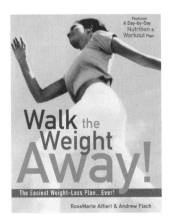
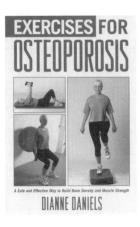
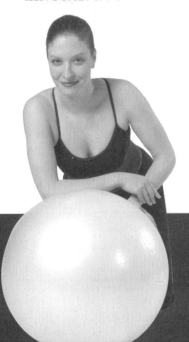

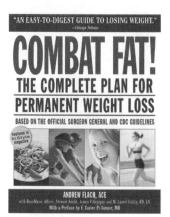
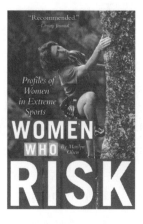
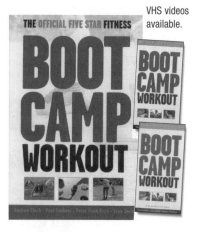

HEALTHY LIVING BOOKS

Healthy Living Books brings together recognized experts from the fields of health, medicine, fitness, and nutrition to provide millions of men and women with the reliable information they need to lead longer, healthier lives.

Our editors recognize that good health comes from healthy lifestyle choices: eating well, exercising regularly, and preventing illness through sound knowledge and intelligent action.

In this day and age, when fewer people are covered by health insurance and more face increased health risks due to sedentary lifestyles, improper nutrition, and the challenges of aging, there is a profound need for solid, tested guidance. That's where we fit in.

Our medical team consists of physicians and specialists from the country's leading medical centers and institutions. Our recipes are kitchen-tested for reliability and include nutritional analysis so that home cooks will find it easy to put delicious, healthful meals on the table. Our exercise programs are prepared by nationally certified personal trainers and rehabilitation experts. All titles are presented in clear, concise language that makes reading fun and useful.

Visit our Web site at www.healthylivingbooks.com

Healthy Living Books has something for everyone.